The Energy of Healing

Edited by Erica Glessing

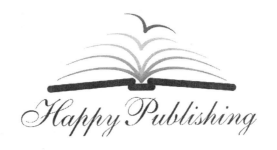

Happy Publishing

The Energy of Healing

Compiled and Edited by Erica Glessing

FIRST EDITION

ISBN: 978-0-9896332-3-9

Cover Design by Melinda Asztalos
Interior Book Design by www.BookPublishingMentor.com

Published by Happy Publishing, www.HappyPublishing.net

Foreword

Dear Reader,

My name is Sadie Lake and I'm a recovering perfectionist. I'll bet you can't relate to that at all. Surely, I'm the only one. Nobody besides me believes they have to prove the rightness of them whilst actually believing they're a big pile of poo.

I have spent most of my life trying to be the best... or at least better. Better than what? Well, better than whatever meager mediocrity I thought I was... anything better than that. I'm just little ol' me; bastard child to a teenage mom, victim of sexual and other abuses, probably not worth the words on this page. I have been well armed to fight this battle called life. I have had so many wounds to heal. Don't you see how damaged I am? No? You're too busy tending your own wounds to notice? Did you slap on a layer of tough armor and go about the business of pretending you were good enough, too?

How has that worked out for you?

For me, it hasn't. But you know what has? The profound

discovery that there was never anything wrong with me in the first place. I can rationalize being the effect of my life: I signed up for this before I came into this world, it's just karma, I needed to learn some powerful lessons.

How about: I AM A POWERFUL CREATOR. Would I like to create more trauma and drama? Or would I like to choose something greater? The healing I've spent my life seeking finally showed up when I acknowledged that no healing was required.

Here is what I have come to know: healing is what happens in the presence of total allowance with absolutely no judgments limiting communion with the oneness and consciousness of all that exists.

When all points of view are removed, whatever had become distorted can return to its optimal state with total ease the way a river flows unhindered when the flood gates of a dam are opened. The universe orients itself to ever and constant expansion with tenacious ferocity, like the way that weeds grow up through concrete sidewalks and parking lots in search of the sun.

The expansion of a blossoming life force will always overcome that which is stagnant and resistant. My armor had created stagnation and resistance to me being me, keeping in place the illusion that what lay beneath was weak, wrong, and vulnerable. Removing the barriers, the judgments, and the need to protect or defend actually allowed me to choose something greater. Life always begets more life. Healing is the energy of the constant expansion of life for the creation of what is greater for the whole... because everything is part of the whole, and everything is whole.

It is interesting how we have used language to separate us from what is most natural for our being. The dictionary defines the word "heal" as to "become whole again". The idea that one requires healing connotes that one has somehow become "not-whole". This is a non-reality. In other words, it's a lie. As the brilliant and wise Albert Einstein said "Energy cannot be created or destroyed, it can only be changed from one form to another." We can never be not-whole. It is our point of view that something is lacking or wrong that creates what we have defined as the necessity for some kind of healing.

With judgment removed, whatever is in discord can return to harmony. It is the polarity, or the "charge" of judgment that disrupts the natural harmony within which all of nature exists. When life is "in flow" there is no resistance. A tree doesn't wish to be a rock. A kidney doesn't wish to be a bone. Just as our body requires that our bones be bones, so that the whole can move and function optimally, the greatness of being exactly what it is, all of life is in harmony. These harmonic states actually create resonant frequencies which invite everything around them into coherence as well. This is the energy of healing: the continual and constant returning to harmony by communion with and contribution to the whole by all of its constituent parts being the greatness of them, unaltered by the presence of judgment.

So how do we create the presence of no judgment? How do we heal? What harmony and healing are the authors of this book offering as a possibility for you? This is what this book, "The Energy of Healing," is inviting you to discover.

Sadie Lake

Table of Contents

Chapter 1

What If You Could See What I See?

By Ashley Stamatinos

Being able to see energy gives you a peek behind the curtain and allows you to see illness or health in people, and to perceive the spirits and guides around us. In addition, you can even feel what exactly is taking place within a body as it is being healed.

I didn't grow up seeing energy; my gift of clairvoyance, or clear seeing, opened up for me when I was 18 years old. At the tender age of 18, I became very ill. After months and months of testing with clinical specialists I was diagnosed with fibromyalgia, chronic pain and chronic fatigue. In fact, I was so sick and depressed that I actually felt like I was dying. It was then, when I hit rock bottom, that my abilities to heal and see energy naturally emerged.

Thankfully, I am now fully healthy and thriving in all areas of my life. No longer do I have the illnesses that once debilitated me to my lowest point. The silver lining perhaps is that out of my illness and depression came many gifts. Out of this struggle I was blessed with the gift of second sight.

My definition of healing has changed drastically over the years. The biggest shift in my understanding of healing is that giving and receiving healing can be much easier than you can imagine. Each exchange of healing energy creates something so beautiful that it's hard to describe with words. Healing takes place all around us all the time. The universe is happy to supply endless reservoirs that you can tap into at any given moment if only you are willing to choose it.

As my gift of seeing the energy world developed, I was able to open up my awareness of what is possible for us. The only way I can illustrate this is by sharing personal examples with you of what I have seen.

I'll never forget it; while I was living in New York City, I vividly remember starting to see energy around me. For example, I would be riding a bus or a train and be overwhelmed as well as captivated by all of the energy I could see glowing from all of the people around me. Close your eyes for a moment and imagine this; a superhighway exchange of light energy flowing back and forth like a steady stream of cars sped up on a reel. Literally, I could see thoughts flying out of people's heads as well as the energy of stress and anxiety buzzing around people. Interestingly enough, I could tell who was sick because their energy would be dull contracted energy. Alternatively, healthy people had vibrant expanded bright energy.

Energy even flows during face-to-face interactions. For example, I noticed that as I was having a conversation with someone where I could actually see who was engaged and who was not interested in what I was sharing with them. The people who were engaged and interested would expand their energy more and more as we spoke. On the other hand, the people who were either confused or not engaged would shrink in their energy.

Within the first year of being able to see energy, I was constantly being asked to look at people's energy and share with them what I saw. One night I was at a friend's home and I'll never forget, a woman in her 40s came into the room I was in, and I dimmed the lights so I could better see her energy. When using this technique, I found that I could see energy better. After all, the energy emitting from us is light, and I could focus better on a person's energy without other lights distracting me. So I took a look at her energy field and could see that there were two big dense balls of energy in her torso area. Feeling a slight reservation, I went on to tell her exactly what I saw as well as where I saw these balls of energy in her body. She paused for a moment. Then took one look at me and with her eye brows raised, informed me that she had two tumors precisely in the exact same two spots where I had pointed out. We both were surprised, to say the least.

To be completely honest, I think my heart skipped a beat because up until that moment I had no idea that I had the ability to see into people's bodies to that degree. I knew nothing about this woman and to have such a huge validation like that was an eye-opening moment. It really stopped me in my tracks and made me realize I that I had the potential to help people with this ability.

As my ability to see energy rapidly started increasing so did the skill of energy healing. One day while I was commuting home I had just stepped off the Long Island Railroad and I walked over to the bus to take me home. As I stood there at the bus stop waiting for the next bus to arrive, I felt something start tingling in the palms of my hands. There was a man next to me who started coughing and looked sick. The heat in my hands increased until I felt like there was a mini fire in each of my palms. It didn't hurt, although it was very intense. Relying on my instincts, I just knew that there was energy coming out of my hands and going to this man who needed healing. Similar situations like that kept happening where my palms heated up around sick people. Yet another sign, so I started to deeply investigate what I could do with this healing ability.

Going about this journey would've been impossible without the love and support of my friends and family. I'm so grateful that I have such wonderful people in my life because when I told my friends about this, they responded by lining up for me to practice energy healing on them. For instance, my friend Jeanette had a bad case of bronchitis. She had chronic bronchitis every year, and she told me it usually lasted for about three months.

At the time, I was living on Long Island and Jeanette was in Manhattan so I instructed her to lie on her couch in her apartment in Manhattan for an hour while I worked on her from Long Island. Energy doesn't have borders or known limits, which is why I was going to give her a remote healing session.

At the time, I imagined her lying on my couch in my apartment, and I stood over the couch as if she was right there in front of me. For an hour, I let energy pour through me, from the universe, and into her. As the energy surged through my hands, my apartment filled up with spirits who helped during the healing process. When I think about it, I must have had about 12 different healing spirits in that room with me all assisting me as I worked on my friend. There was so much energy from the healing and from all the spirits in the room that the temperature in the room dropped and was freezing. This happens quite often when there are spirits in a room with you.

As I looked at the couch, I could see her energy as clearly as if she was laying there. I could see the imbalances in her lungs as dark fuzzy strands of energy. Then I continued to look at her energy for signs that the session was complete. So I swept my hands over her energy a few times and was looking for the once bumpy energy to feel smoothed out. Once I felt her energy was smooth and her lungs looked healed, I called her on the phone and told her the session was over and she could move around now.

Jeanette called me in the morning to tell me how she was

feeling. Much to my delight, when she called me she excitedly reported that her cough was gone and she felt great! She reminded me that she usually had the bronchitis for months, and this was very noticeable that she felt so much better. She continued to touch base with me regularly and could see the constant positive progression in her lungs. I'm thrilled to say that the bronchitis didn't return that year again.

These occurrences sparked something inside of me. I found energy healing incredibly fascinating and started taking classes in order to obtain certifications in as many different healing modalities I could find. With this knowledge, I wanted to learn how I could use these skills and abilities to heal myself as well as anyone who desired my healing services.

When I first started working with energy, I started doing hands-on energy healing. At that point, my definition of energy healing only included where one person gave the other person energy through mentally sending the energy or physically laying on of hands. This was really just the very beginning of my healing journey.

Later on, my definition of healing developed into something much more expansive where I learned to connect with the universe in a deeper way. Typically, I ask the universe to increase my capacity for healing where the power of asking the universe questions really increased my ability to send healing energy and to see what else was taking place during a healing session.

During my pregnancy, my son helped me to expand my awareness of what is possible with healing energy. While I was pregnant I had a deep knowing that my child was connected to the universe in a different way then what I was familiar with.

Even when I was pregnant with my son, I always gave him a sense of choice. I never automatically gave him energy healing, I always asked if he wanted me to channel healing to him. When he said yes, I would go through a list of all the modalities I had learned and ask him what he would like me to send to him. He would tell me he didn't want any of them.

It was so interesting to me that he didn't want to receive any of the modalities I had learned. (If you haven't already guessed, I was telepathically speaking with my unborn child). He told me that he was an evolved being, and that his energy was vibrating at such a fast frequency that all of the modalities that I knew were simply too slow for him. Of course this made me smile as he told me this. There I was, thinking about how advanced I was because I achieved a level of mastery in many healing modalities, and my son's messages helped me to uncover what's possible with healing beyond what I knew.

As I started to work with my son when he said yes to healing, I'd put my hands on my belly and ask him to allow me to be a channel for him. I told him to pull whatever energy he desired through me and he could receive whatever it was that he knew was in vibrational alignment with what he required. This worked for both of us because I simply put my ego aside (including any thoughts about what I thought he needed), and I allowed myself to simply observe the process.

What I found fascinating was that I could feel exactly when he pulled energy through me. This new awareness indicated that this energy was derived from other planets that were not on any charts I had seen. He showed me where he was pulling energy from, and it looked like a planet that had electric blue light filling it. It was absolutely beautiful. As I channeled this energy to him it felt like a twinkling feeling in my body. The energy was moving at such a high frequency that it felt like it was tickling me as I channeled it.

He would suck up the energy so fast that sometimes my hands only needed to be on my belly giving him that energy for two or three minutes. He had no conclusions or definitions about how long a session needed to be. He didn't need a half an hour session or an hour session or a two hour session because he literally would pull everything he required within a couple minutes.

After that experience with my son, it hit me...I had an another ah ha moment where I realized so much more is possible when it comes to healing our bodies and our lives. Along this journey, I looked at all the definitions I had created about how healing needed to be given or received, and chose to completely let go of all of them.

When we choose to receive healing for ourselves, this can

actually be the greatest source of giving to those closest to us. I've heard so many of my clients who are Empaths tell me that they feel guilty taking time for themselves. What I'd like to illustrate for you is that choosing to care for yourself isn't selfish. In fact, it can actually unlock and heal those around you simply by choosing to work on yourself.

An example of this is was when I came home from a master-level healing course where I had received multiple energy activations. I was feeling like I was on cloud nine. My sheer level of excited drew my husband in for a conversation on the couch. As he sat on the couch, I began to share what I learned with my husband. Shortly after we started chatting, he started feeling so relaxed around me that he fell asleep by 7:30 pm (and that's very rare for him).

When you change your energy and change your vibration like I did in that class, the people around you will feel it too. Basically, you can imagine that if we are made of energy, our energy expands and upgrades after a healing class or session, and the people who are closest to us will receive healing by being near you.

This can often look like physical healing, but you might also unlock their judgments or help them release their feelings of depression or low self-esteem. It's often so obvious, that the person around you will seem different overnight. This was the case with my husband. The next morning when he woke up he felt like a million bucks. He asked me if I did some kind of healing or attunement on him because he felt really wonderful. I simply smiled and explained that I didn't purposely do anything, I only worked on myself, and that choice to work on myself had contributed to him in a big way.

Because I gave up all my definitions of healing, I started seeing shifts take place. I realized that as I walked into a grocery store if I asked my body to soak in all of the nutrients and vitamins that it required to receive healing, my body would actually receive what it required. I also taught my child to do the same thing by putting pictures in his head to show him how to soak in anything needed to fill any areas of depletion.

When I do this, I start to feel high as my body receives everything it needs. It feels like it is buzzing. It's kind of like the feeling you get right after a deep meditation or after walking out of a great yoga class, or from having a great massage.

What this new awareness did for me was it allowed me to walk through my life in a way that I was receiving healing throughout my day all the time without having to sit down on my couch and put my hands on my body for a set amount of time. As my life became busier, that kind of structure was too limiting for me. I'm moving a million miles a minute all the time in my life and I needed to find a way that I could work with energy healing so that it contributed to me and I was able to keep moving fast. I needed to allow myself to be filled up consistently with energy so that I could continue to be as busy as I desired without getting burnt out.

Now I walk through life asking the sky, the earth, all of the molecules and everything around me to contribute to me. I open myself up to receive the energy all around me that would like to gift to me. It's as simple as opening yourself up to this and choosing it. I'm all about making things easier and not over complicating this. You don't need to get into your head and figure this out. Just open yourself up and receive.

These energy exchanges occur throughout every moment of my life. This is usually a quiet conversation that I'm having, in my mind, with the molecules around me, asking them to contribute to me. It may sound wacky to you, however it has given me unlimited sustainable energy, and opened doors for me that I have never opened before. It's as if I'm an energizer bunny being constantly filled up with endless reservoirs of energy, which is probably why so many people have told me that what I accomplish in a day they don't accomplish in a week.

Imagine just for a moment that you were able to tap into this type of healing? How would that contribute to your life? What would it feel like if you could receive unlimited sustainable energy? Would it change anything? Please understand that energy has no boundaries and no limits, which means that you have the capacity to impact the trajectory of your life and those around you if you choose it.

About the Author

ASHLEY STAMATINOS

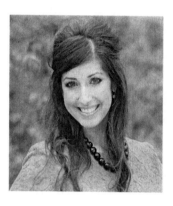

Ashley is a co-author of the #1 bestselling book "The Energy of Expansion", and is widely known as the Empath Expert for her extensive work with highly sensitive adults and children. She has been interviewed on TV multiple times for her work with sensitive people. Her mission is to empower you to use your sensitivity as your greatest strength.

Ashley is the founder of Omorfi Healing, a business that she created as a platform to offer holistic education and healing to the world. She is passionate about teaching, and has been teaching for the last 10+ years. Many of her students have said that Ashley teaches with great patience and enthusiasm.

Within her practice she offers both online and in-person courses to those seeking a life they love. Her in-person courses are primarily available within the Chicagoland area at premier energy education centers.

While Ashley's main focus within her practice is supporting highly sensitive people, she also has many other courses available for you. She teaches on a variety of topics. Some of the courses she teaches include: How to Communicate with Spirits, A new Perspective on Parenting Intuitive Children, Empowering Holistic Teachers, Ignite Your Holistic Practice, Seeing and Knowing The Bioenergetic Field, Mediumship Development, Empowering The Empath and Powering Up Empathic Kids to list a few.

Ashley had just moved to NYC days before 9/11, and shortly thereafter she developed severe fibromyalgia, chronic fatigue, chronic pain and a piercing lung infection.

As a result, she was placed on powerful medications (including epileptic seizure medication) for years until she reached rock bottom. It came to a point where she was so sick that she felt like she was dying. Unfortunately, western medications were not helping, so she started exploring other avenues of treatment when she stumbled upon alternative modalities of treatment.

Immediately, there was a shift and a transformation that was occurring within Ashley. Her health started to improve rapidly to the shock of her doctors. As her journey of personal healing took off like a rocket, she began to see the world in a different light. Finally, she was able to feel relief and realize what it truly meant to live a fulfilling life.

Because of her personal healing experience, it led her to her calling of teaching holistic wellness and empowerment courses. Miraculously, Ashley has eliminated all symptoms and leads a very different life now. One that is full of purpose, passion and optimum health in all areas of life.

She feels her real "credentials" have come from personally overcoming and conquering these health battles. Now, Ashley openly shares her recipe for healing the incurable from her unique perspective about overcoming life's obstacles.

Wondering if you're an Empath? Take the free Am I an Empath? Quiz on the home page of Ashley's website.

Wondering if you have undiscovered Psychic skills? Take the free What is My Psychic Gift? Quiz on the home page of Ashley's website.

Private one-on-one phone sessions are also available for you. You can go to her website and click on Private Sessions to get all of the details.

Ashley does travel to guest lecture, and teach her specialty classes. If you'd like her to come to your business to teach a course or to give a guest lecture, please email info@omorfihealing.com for further information or

Get Social with Ashley:

Facebook.com/OmorfiHealing

YouTube.com/OmorfiHealing

Pinterest.com/OmorfiHealing

www.OmorfiHealing.com

Chapter 2

Moving Beyond the Invisible Cage of Abuse

By Dr. Lisa Cooney, LMFT

"Can you give me the details of your early childhood abuse?"

There was a long silence after my editor asked me this question. She had recently reviewed the first draft of my book, "Kick Abuse in the Caboose," and wanted to fill in more details of my past.

I asked her to give me a moment so I could summon up my past abuse. It took eight minutes for me to begin listing the details to her. During those eight minutes I scanned my body, amazed to discover that the two decades of physical, sexual, emotional, financial, spiritual and physiological abuse I had experienced no longer inhabited my body.

As I shared the details with her I felt as if I was sharing a client's or a friend's story, not mine. I wasn't dissociating or disconnecting. I had become the embodiment of one who has healed and transcended abuse.

I smiled as I realized how far I had come in my journey of moving beyond abuse.

I remember feeling the heaviness of the perpetration. I read dozens of self-help books and highlighted sentences until the words leapt off the page and entered me, giving me a glimpse of a different reality. Knowing that others understood what I was experiencing gave me hope. I wasn't alone.

I tried to hike, meditate, swim and bike the abuse out of me. I sought counseling, and even earned a Master's degree and a Doctorate in Psychology myself. I was committed to continually educating myself clinically, energetically and psychologically. I was determined to find a way to move beyond abuse.

As I facilitated workshop after workshop and freed others from their abuse I ultimately freed myself as well. I have committed my life to eradicating and eliminating abuse in all its many forms from this planet through the Beyond Abuse Revolution.

Moving Beyond Abuse: A New Paradigm of Healing

Perhaps you have experienced abuse. The abuse may have been sexual, physical, spiritual, financial or emotional and it could have taken the form of a single event or a series of incidents.

You may have already invested a vast amount of time and energy in healing your experience of abuse. Perhaps you have not seen the results you desired. I have found that a lot of tools and practices that preceded the approach I take to moving beyond abuse are about fixing ourselves and defining ourselves by our story of abuse.

The therapy model especially teaches us that we must fix ourselves in order to be free. When we adopt this model, we assume that there is something wrong with us and we look for solutions to fix the problem. It becomes a bottomless pit. We never get to the end of it because we never feel fixed or whole. You may have found yourself going around in similar circles, wondering if it will ever end; waiting for the day when you are finally healed.

This chapter (which is an excerpt from my upcoming book, "Kick Abuse In The Caboose") turns the old paradigm of dealing with abuse on its head. You are going to discover that you do not need to fix anything or remain defined by your abuse. You will discover how to make the choice of ending perpetration and no longer allowing that one act or series of events to dominate your entire life.

The Invisible Cage of Abuse

I spent much of my life in an invisible cage.

I say it was invisible because although I lived inside it, a silent prisoner, I wasn't even aware that it existed. It took me decades to name it, let alone to shape it into a message that I could share with the world. Yet every time I talk about the invisible cage to someone who has experienced abuse, a look of recognition, often relief, sweeps across their face. You may be having a similar experience yourself right now as you read these words.

The cage includes a subtle judgment about the wrongness of you that you take for granted to be true. In other words, you perceive yourself to be bad or wrong because of the abuse that occurred. This "wrongness" becomes the filter through which you experience and perceive reality. You create your life from the perpetration and imprison yourself within it.

Your cage is like a ghost that continuously whispers in your ear. It whispers when you have challenges. Yet when life is good, it doesn't stop. In fact, at these times it is likely to get louder with a desperate attempt to keep you inside the cage of abuse. Living within the limits of the cage keeps you held in a place that is familiar. There is a strange comfort in the confines of the cage, however much you desire to live beyond it.

The cage is based on lack, limitation and lie.

The cage keeps you out of freedom, pleasure and possibility.

To live inside the cage is to live without a voice. You may be able to speak and function in the world, but there is a part of you that is isolated, silenced and cut off from reality. A part that lives inside you, deadened and numbed out.

The pain of living inside the cage can be so great that sometimes you choose not to dwell there at all. You may numb out or check out to avoid the pain. You might do this periodically throughout the day, checking out of your body. You may also use food, alcohol, drugs or medication to check out more deeply. You become a shell of who you truly are.

You wonder why you are 'self-sabotaging', when what you are actually doing is operating from what the cage is designed to do: fight life and say 'no' from a place of contraction rather than embrace life and say 'yes' from a place of expansion. Inside the cage you continue to react to life from the patterns of past abuse. This keeps the perpetration alive.

You may have also noticed that when you live from within the cage of abuse, it reverberates through all other areas of your life. When you are filtering the world through the lens of abuse, more of it is drawn to you. This can lead to more self-blame. Maybe you have heard phrases such as, 'You create your own reality,' and when the pattern of abuse continuously perpetuates itself and you don't know how to stop it, it adds to the feeling that there is something wrong with you.

What I have often seen happen from within the cage is that because abuse mires our reality, often our perception gets twisted into a mild form of insanity. What seems true can be false and vice versa. We find ourselves trusting people who shouldn't be trusted, and not trusting people who we could. People may come into our lives that represent all the things we have been saying we want to generate and manifest, but we push them away because to engage with them would mean living beyond the cage and we feel uncomfortable doing so.

If you have been walking around in the invisible cage of abuse, up until now you've probably assumed that this was your only choice. In fact, for most people that I have worked with, the idea of choice at first seems confusing. We have been sold the myth that because we have experienced abuse our lives will be forever filled with suffering. Your life, up until now, has possibly provided you with plenty of evidence that this is the case.

Yet living in the invisible cage of abuse as a silent prisoner is not your only choice.

Make Friends with the Cage of Abuse

What I have discovered in supporting tens of thousands of people around the world to overcome abuse is that we don't necessarily make our way out of the cage by a quick fix. First we increase our awareness and acknowledge the cage.

In this moment you may be waking up for the first time to understanding that the cage exists. I often hear people say, "Oh, that's what it is," when they hear me talk about the cage. We are giving words to something that usually remains unnamed.

I often say it's like there has been an elephant shitting in the room all along and everyone was silently stepping around it. We are no longer ignoring it. It stinks, and we are dealing with it.

After you acknowledge the cage you get to accept the cage that you've been living in. The cage has actually been your biggest ally in healing: it protected you during a time you needed protection.

When you embrace the cage and choose something other than shutting down, you soften. You open to the possibility of being in communion with your pain. This is ultimately the only way to dissolve the bars of the cage and step into true freedom.

When you make friends with the cage of abuse you connect with the freedom, joy and possibility that exists independent of the cage. In order to step out of the cage you don't actually have to get anything back. This is where my approach differs radically from what you may have experienced before. Instead, you learn how to make different kinds of choices that don't perpetuate the abuse. You discover how to connect with yourself beyond the insanity that created the cage in the first place.

And you choose to live without making what happened to you (whether it was a single act or a series of events) into your entire life.

It is likely that your whole reality will begin to shift as you start to notice how the invisible cage shows up in your own life.

Moving Beyond The Cage Of Abuse

The cruel joke about abuse is that it ended a long time ago yet you keep it going by treating yourself like the abuser treated you. Why do you do this?

The invisible cage of abuse holds you prisoner to the belief that you are somehow wrong or bad; that you don't deserve to live for yourself but rather need to do what others think you should do, or what you're supposed to do (just like what happened during your abuse: you did what you were told and your needs didn't matter).

As you make friends with the cage of abuse you stop being at war with yourself. This is the place from which you start choosing you and committing to your own life.

What does it look like to commit to your own life?

Committing to your life looks like standing up for what you choose no matter what happens. It's never giving in and never giving up (says the Irish Fighter in me). And yet it's not about pushing, efforting, excluding or fighting.

You no longer need to prove or fight to have your life for yourself. You simply get to choose it. This commitment to life is not heavy – it's actually the ease, lightness, joy and fun that's possible when you choose for you. And it actually requires a kindness with yourself that you may never have experienced before.

What is the biggest block to committing to you?

I've guided thousands of people to overcome their sexual abuse and one of the biggest challenges I see them struggle with is letting go of their story of abuse. It's their story, and the role of victim within the story, that keeps them from committing to themselves.

It's like they were more committed to the story of abuse rather than the possibility of life beyond it. I've been there myself. I know this. Yet it only needs to be a "phase" in your journey from the cage of abuse to radical aliveness.

What happens when you hold onto the story of abuse?

When you hold onto the story of abuse you keep yourself trapped in the role of "victim." It seems like "life happens" to you; that you are a victim of circumstance; that no matter what you do you're going to get f*cked anyway, so why bother?

Abuse becomes a great excuse for not committing to your own life.

I'm here to show you there is another possibility. When you put down the story of abuse, when you get support to release all the inner anguish about your abuse, you open up space for something new.

What's possible when you commit to your own life?

As you move out of the cage of abuse and the wrongness of you, you discover the phenomenance of you. You become radically alive: a space of being where the abuse no longer runs your life and you are generating and creating a life for yourself far beyond anything you could have ever imagined.

About the Author

DR. LISA COONEY, LMFT

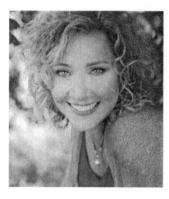

Dr. Lisa Cooney is a leading authority on thriving after childhood sexual abuse. As a licensed Marriage and Family Therapist, certified Access Consciousness Facilitator, Master Theta Healer and #1 bestselling author in the books "The Energy of Happiness," "The Energy of Receiving," "The Energy of Expansion" and author of the upcoming books, "Kick Abuse in the Caboose: The Bridge to Radical Aliveness" and "When Did You Become a Slave to Abuse: Getting Free in a New Way."

She has supported thousands of people over the past 20 years move beyond their abuse to create infinite possibilities for themselves and joyful lives. Find her at www.DrLisaCooney.com.

To find more tools and resources for moving beyond abuse and into radical aliveness please visit: www.DrLisaCooney.com.. You can also join the weekly radio show, "Beyond Abuse, Beyond Therapy, Beyond Anything."

Stay tuned for updates as to when "Kick Abuse In The Caboose" will be available. Commit to you. Join the Beyond Abuse Revolution.

Chapter 3

From Broken to Beautiful

By Minette the Energist

Would you be open to the possibility that our bodies can heal quickly, easily and in some cases instantaneously? Would you allow it, accept it, believe it? In truth, our bodies are amazing and intelligent and are designed to heal themselves. This healing system exists within us and is waiting for us to activate it with the right space and energy.

Our bodies know what they need better than anyone else. They know what is needed for healing to take place. If we listen. Our bodies communicate to us daily about everything. Alas, in this reality we are not taught to listen to our bodies, to check in and say "Hi, Body How Are you doing today?" It's when we do not listen and we ignore our body that the beginning of the dis "ease" path in the body starts. I share with you my journey from broken to beautiful and what I have learned about the Energy of Healing.

A painful experience can be the most beautiful healing journey, and mine started when I slipped and fell. (A mentor told me, I chose this awakening to reconnect to the awareness's I had been suppressing.) This choice lead me on a painful journey as it took a year for doctors to find out my neck was broken. By this time, my internal organs had begun to shutdown, I had been hospitalized several times and even put into the ICU cardiac unit (because apparently having the amount of chest pain that comes from a broken neck can look like a cardiac incident). Here my body was put through test after test; x-rays, cat scans, a cardiac stress test, EKG's and an angiogram but nothing was found. I had excruciating pain, headaches and limited use of my left hand. It wasn't until a caring doctor listened to me when I told him that something was wrong with my body. He took another look at my medical history and noticed no one ever ordered an MRI after my fall. An MRI was ordered and it revealed that my neck was broken. I was immediately sent to a surgeon, who after viewing my MRI asked "if I had been skydiving without a parachute?" Then he said I needed immediate surgery and that he did not even know how I was walking around. He told me, that if I even bumped my head I would be paralyzed from the neck down. (This was shocking and terrifying, but at the same time a strange relief to know what was wrong). So the day after Christmas I had the surgery. They removed the broken bones and replaced them with a titanium cage, plates and screws. I was told it would take about 2 years to recover. Now I was left to deal with all the damage that had been done to my body from my prolonged injury. The doctors cut out a piece of my intestine and then started talking about cutting out my liver and gallbladder....My body screamed "NO!!! ENOUGH!!" It woke me. I had never felt my body scream like this. I could hear it weeping like a child. It was in that moment, I knew something else had to be possible.

So after more than a year of suffering in this medical reality, I took responsibility for my own healing. I made the choice and had an awareness of my body's energy that I had never known before.

Reconnecting with my body

I began to follow this new energy. I felt a level of communication with my body developing. I had the awareness my body was upset with me for not listening for so long, for being disconnected for so long. So I started with pep talks to my body saying "we can heal", "we can do anything" which helped but it was not enough. I had another awareness that my body wanted more. You see I had loved myself but never took the time to tell my body how much I loved it. So I began to tell my body how much it was loved and appreciated. How I now realized, everything that it had done for me and everything it had allowed me to do; every breath it had taken, every tear it had shed, every step it had taken, every time it had bled.

I asked myself, "Could it be this easy?" And for me this first shift was easy. I could feel a change in the energy. I had an even greater level of awareness of my body. I was aware how much my body still loved me, even though I had neglected to return this love until now. I embraced the attitude of gratitude. I thanked my body for everything; allowing me to create life, allowing me to walk, to talk, eyes to see, arms to hug, lips to kiss, hands to hold. The more gratitude I expressed to my body the more the energy flowed with ease. From this space of gratitude I started to create new possibilities for healing.

Creating the space to heal

"We limit our bodies healing capacities. Our point of view creates our reality. If we think we are sick, we are sick. If we know we can heal, we can heal. We must clear the heaviness of negative emotions, they are very destructive. They rob us of joy, love and happiness and we need these positive energies for healing. We are capable of creating an energetic shift in our bodies. We must first create a space where this is possible, where the energy of healing can fill our bodies. This space is expansive and light, where miracles can happen."

Mind, Body and Spirit

As I reconnected to my body, I started my healing with the physical body and meeting its needs for nourishment and movement. I began taking supplements and vitamins. I was still however in a lot of pain. When I experienced pain, I noticed the heaviness and contraction I felt. I even contracted my breath. So I began choosing not to go into heaviness and contract or put up energetic barriers. I took conscious breaths expanding my body. I choose to express gratitude for this awareness of intensity in my body. I would do energetic exercises where I would expand my awareness out 100 miles which made the intensity lessen for me. I checked in daily with my body. "Body, do you need anything? what would you like to eat? to wear? to do?". I learned how to muscle test. Which was a very useful tool, it allowed me another way to communicate with my body. This new level of communion with my body was fantastic. I could feel energy flowing even stronger.

I became a student of energy. I studied different energy healing modalities. I became a practitioner of Access Consciousness Bars & Body Processes, N.L.P, E.F.T, Thetahealing, Reiki and Seraphim Angel. They all taught energy and how to shift, clear or change it. They taught me more of the mind, body and spirit aspect of healing. I knew my mind was impacting my healing but I had not realized to what degree. I knew sending love and gratitude to my body was helping to lighten the energy and help it flow. But this was just the start.

I started to heal the effects my mind had on my body. I identified everywhere my body felt heavy, or carried energies or emotions that made me feel heavy. Anger was a big one for me. I had people who had hurt me terribly in my life. So I started with forgiveness. I forgave everyone who had hurt me. I've had some people ask how I forgave so easily and it's because I was not doing it for them, I was doing it for me and my body's healing. Holding on to anger only hurts the one who holds onto it. I forgave myself for not lis-tening to my body, and for all the poor choices I had made with stress, food, exercise, relationships and anything else I had done. I forgave the doctors who put me thru so much. I forgave l and began making conscious choices. Fear was another heaviness I was carrying. I worked at identifying my fears and clearing them. I replaced these heavy negative thoughts with positive light ones. I began focusing on what my body healing would feel like to me and how my body being healed would make me feel, what I would do when my body was healed. I envisioned hiking with my family, bending to smell the flowers and swimming in the ocean and what the waves would feel like against my body. These visions filled me with joy and added to the beautiful space of healing I was creating. I became conscious and aware of my words. Words are very powerful and have energy. I stopped saying "I will fight this", as this energy seemed to bring up a heaviness for me, like that of a battle. I did not want to fight anything. I only desired the energy of communion and contribution with my body. I started saying "I am healing" instead of "I will heal" as these brought up very different energies for me as well. As I continued to do this it became easier and easier to follow the energy and what my body was telling me.

The final healing for me was that of my spirit. I realized my connection to Source (Creator of all that is). I knew I was not alone, and that I was connected to everyone and every-thing. This feeling of oneness was beyond belief. I perceived energy of ease, love and peace. I felt this sense of everything wanting to contribute to my healing. So I began to tap into that energy. I started giving and receiving love from the earth, the flowers, trees, birds, universe and so much more. I connected in ways I never thought possible. I was whole and complete. It is magical having my mind, body and spirit be connected in the space of who I truly BE.

Oneness

It is in this space of oneness and ease, that I found the energy for true healing. I had a new frequency and vibration that was phenomenal. This higher frequency immediately started attracting amazing individuals into my life, doctors, scientists, energy workers. I began to attract people who are working to create a new energetic healing reality.

Things to remember:

1. Start your day with gratitude.

At least once every morning and evening list 5 things you are grateful for. The more often you express gratitude the better the energy flows. (Science has proven that a grateful heart is good for you. That gratitude positively affects your heart and nervous system, which in turn aids your immune function, reduces stress, anxiety, sadness, insomnia and so much more.) And since stress contributes to sickness and the dis"ease" path in our bodies, isn't it time we made a choice, to stop contributing to this dis"ease path of our own bodies and started choosing gratitude to develop the energy and space for healing.)

2. Honor your body every day.

At least once every morning and evening tell your body 5 things you love about it and 5 things that you appreciate that it does or allows you to do. Feel how the energy changes in your body.

3. Communicate with your body.

Listen to and check in with your body throughout the day. "Hi, body. How are you? Do you need anything? What would you like to eat?"

4. Create a space of healing by clearing negative energies and replacing them with positive ones.

Clear heavy (low frequency) energies like anger, guilt, regret and fear from your body. Forgive others including yourself. Invite in love, joy and happiness (high frequencies) to take their place.

Every healthy cell has a frequency and when this frequency is disrupted by low frequencies, the cell becomes abnormal. So when we restore this healthy high frequency the cell can be healed.

5. Connect to your higher self and who you truly BE!!

Love yourself and know that you are loved. Know that you are worthy of being healed. You are connected to everything. Know how much the earth and universe want to contribute to you and what a contribution you are. Hold your highest vibrational frequency and just BE with total ease and joy.

Thank you for being part of my journey from broken to beautiful and how I started to create the energy and space for my own healing. My journey continues everyday and my body is my Best friend. How does it get any better than that!? And everyday day it surprises me because it keeps getting better. Here's to everyone helping to create a new energetic healing reality, full of infinite possibilities, magic and miracles.

About the Author
MINETTE THE ENERGIST

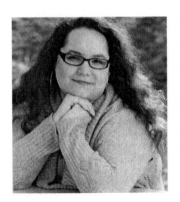

My name is Minette Sanchez, also known as the Internal Energist. I am a certified professional life coach, Energy Worker, Access Consciousness® Certified Bars Practitioner and Facilitator as well as an Access Consciousness® Certified Body Process Facilitator, radio show host, motivational speaker, and author, with a background in business and psychology. I am the proud owner of Internal Energies, a company whose goal is to help people create more ease, joy, and possibilities in all aspects of their life (relationships, finances, body, etc.).

I was born in California and have been blessed with an Amazing husband Eric, who I have had the joy and pleasure of creating the last 25 years of my life with and looking forward to many more. We have two sweet, kind, highly intelligent and beautiful daughters; Ashlyn and Jocelyn. I am filled with gratitude and so much love for my AMAZING family, whose love and support has allowed me to go on this beautiful journey. I am also so grateful and filled with joy for this amazing life I am living, and enjoy everyday getting to share that joy with my clients and helping them create more happiness and possibilities in their lives as well. As an Internal Energist, I get to assist people daily in creating and finding ways to enjoy more ease with their bodies, I am trained to perform and teach over 50 different energetic body processes as well as coaching clients to achieve more of what they desire in their life with family, children, work, finances and so much more. So, if you are ready to create more joy and ease in your life or body, visit www.internalenergies.com

Chapter 4

The Healing Road to Home

By Tamara Younker

Home. It could be a physical location somewhere on the planet. Though that's not what I'm referring to when I speak of the healing road to home. For me, healing is continually cultivating an intimacy of being that I now know as home. Intimacy of being is dissolving all barriers to communion with the energy and space of consciousness beyond the definitions and limitations of any carefully constructed mental identity. Why would anyone choose that?

Dr. Dain Heer, co-creator of Access Consciousness®, once said, "Space is not emptiness. Space is the ripeness of every possibility ready to explode when you ask for it." That's the space, the intimacy of being, I aim to function as in every moment. Here everything is a choice available to me, and possibility seems to flourish in a magically unobstructed way. It's not a place. It's a space and in this intimacy of being, I'm home.

Once upon a time...

Once upon a time, a being arrived on beautiful planet Earth and was gifted a body. She was invited to play in this paradise, and delighted in the exploration of this magnificent world. Joy was natural to her as she splashed in mud puddles after the rain, chased butterflies in the tall grass and was caressed by the warmth of the sun on her skin. She wanted to experiment with everything that came into her world. She lived without the weight of any reasons or justifications yielding fully to her insistent desire to simply explore and create. Every action was inspired by the pleasure and enjoyment of being. Life was beautiful, and she was happy.

Wait. That seems like an idyllic childhood, but it wasn't mine.

The childhood I remember was tempered with cruelty. My parents, like most people, functioned from judgment as their primary operating system. My environment was filled with contempt, disapproval, force, criticism, shaming and perhaps the most prominent was the perpetual threat of impending separation by rejection when not performing up to rigid expectations. Though it's not widely acknowledged as such yet, I would call that abusive.

The natural joy of being was not allowed, much less welcome. So, what's a being to do? Withdraw, and wait patiently to be invited into presence again when a more nurturing environment becomes available.

With being in retreat, my mind and sharp intellect took over and became a life preserver. I had to figure out how to survive in this unforgiving environment that felt too brutal for the gentleness of being to remain without being crushed under the demanding boot of judgment.

The control structure of reward and punishment became the landscape to navigate, and learning the rules of right and wrong was top priority in order to avoid the pervasive threat of wrongness and exclusion. Alignment and agreement seemed crucial to survival. This is the reality judgment creates, where being is seemingly cast aside as inconsequential and forgotten, in the attempt to raise good children into right and appropriate rule-following adults.

It didn't take long before I realized rule following didn't appeal to me. So, I became an under-the-radar rebel of magnitude. Alignment and agreement was out, and resistance and reaction was the new mode of operation. Both equally squeeze out any possibility for the presence of being, and solidify an incapacity for freedom. In both, trying to prove I was good and could fit in well with a rule-driven consensus reality, and then fighting against it because I felt entirely powerless in the face of it, I subjugated being in favor of the supremacy of a reality I imagined was greater than being.

It was a lie. But, I bought it. With every choice to invoke

and perpetuate the illusion of my wrongness and power-lessness, I abandoned communion with being.

The natural peace, ease and joyful space of being is lost when we unwittingly isolate from being in favor of role playing. As I progressively divorced being day by day, I carefully constructed a mental fabrication of identity in its place. Judgment, which I learned to master so well in order to function effectively within the confines of consensus reality, was the glue that held the illusion together. The very source of everything I fought against–judgment–paradoxically became my jailer. I succumbed to its Mobius strip of addiction, feeling defenseless and powerless in the face of it, while at the same time feeling dependent on it for control. I solidified my own incapacity for freedom by subjecting myself to the lie of judgment as a source of defense and power.

This incapacity for freedom is perpetuated by the control structure of good versus bad and right versus wrong. It is a recipe for misery. Adopting the mental construct of judgment as a necessary source of power to function and survive in consensus reality abandons being, and the isolation of that separation feels very real.

I refer to that separation from, and isolation of being, as a primary trauma. Freedom of being is abandoned. Nobody did it to me. I chose it, however unwittingly. What it took me a lifetime to realize was that I could choose again. The initial choice to survive utilizing the scaffolding of judgment can be changed. Intimacy of being can be deliberately cultivated by allowing consciousness to thrive in our lives when functioning with awareness.

Discovering Infinite Being

I discovered Access Consciousness® in 2010, and it was then that a whole new world began opening up to me. All I had known to be "real" began to shift and change. I began weaning myself off of the control structures of consensus reality, and began choosing into the space of functioning as an infinite being. In this space, I realize I can have total choice and am no longer bound by the interpretations of right or wrong, good or bad. I stop working hard to prevent things I don't want to happen. I stop trying to control my external environment in an attempt to avoid feeling what I don't want to feel.

This taste of freedom is sweet.

I delight in knowing my superpower of choice allows me to be the sovereign of a reality where possibility prevails. In this space of infinite possibility, there is no scarcity of choice and there is no such thing as a wrong choice. Trusting my awareness and what I know becomes the cornerstone of an undefended confidence unrelated to anything in a judgment-bound consensus reality. I live less and less at the effect of anything and know that life is not happening to me, but rather that I am creating it all. Judgment as a strategy for living has ceased to be relevant to me, and simply becomes obsolete in its usefulness. I claim freedom to function as an infinite being through liberation from the limited constructs of a defined identity and a consensus reality designed only for control.

As I unravel the illusion of judgment, I discover being that has always been present but unattended to in favor of the thoughts, feelings and emotions that serve as the orienting principles of identity. When judgment is no longer operational, communion is natural.

Choice by choice by choice by choice, I create a new reality through cultivating intimacy of being. Infinite being is the oneness and consciousness of all things. Nothing is excluded. With the acknowledgment that I am the sovereign of a reality of my choosing, any self-imposed prison is dissolved into a playground of possibility where something greater can be created beyond anything that currently exists.

Choice Creates

Most of my life I didn't acknowledge the gift of choice and its capacity to create. This refusal is a rejection of the wealth of choice and freedom of an infinite being. I may not have deliberately disavowed choice. I convinced myself I was powerless by interpreting the circumstances of my life as beyond my control. I believed I didn't have a choice, or that there were forces far more powerful than me making my choices for me. That belief anchored me into a position as victim. Consensus reality and all who colluded with it were my perpetrators.

I renounced the freedom and potency of choice in favor of judgment as protection thinking it would give me the power

I needed for survival. That unwitting choice created a life of misery and suffering feeling isolated, alienated, alone, separate and depressed.

Healing separation from being required I claim choice as my greatest generative and creative superpower. Knowing I have choice at my disposal in every moment allows me to advance into the creation of my life rather than retreat from everything I used to avoid. Choice fostered a sense of command as an infinite being, and I realized any earlier need or necessity to control my external environment seemed absurd.

The Imprisonment of Blame

Gary Douglas, the Founder of Access Consciousness®, once delivered to me what we in Access fondly call a "wedgie," a bulls-eye in a blind spot. He asked, "When are you going to stop making yourself so miserable?" Like a seasoned marksman, he hit his target with precision and I was left dumbfounded by the idea that I could be the source of my misery. That question changed my life, and I will be forever grateful.

Blaming someone or something else for the misery I experienced was one of the biggest lies I perpetrated upon myself. Blame requires judgment, and abdicates choice. I must make someone else, something else or myself wrong in order to suffer the self-imposed misery of blame. Blame hijacks being by interpreting events through the construct of judgment.

Judgment is the root of all trauma and drama. By blaming and refusing to acknowledge my choice in creating the trauma and drama in my life, I solidified my point of view that I was at the effect of situations, circumstances, other people and even my own thoughts, feelings and emotions.

Blame is seductive. It establishes a dependency on judgment by perpetuating the lie of wrongness and fault, as well as, serving as effective evidence for the appearance of powerlessness. Releasing blame is healing. When I stopped blaming, the potency of choice was ignited and decades of feeling despair and helplessness vanished.

Healing the Coffins of Conclusion

Most of my life, I had a self-obsessed orientation to the world where I interpreted everything others did to be entirely about me. I made what they did, or didn't do, mean something about me and I formulated stories to support those conclusions gathering evidence everywhere to prove they were true.

I formed conclusions based on how I interpreted the events and circumstances of my early life, and those conclusions became facts about what was real and true. I interpreted my parent's neglect to mean they didn't care about me, and that conclusion ensured that the reality I created was filtered entirely through that point of view. From that interpretation, I constructed seemingly countless coffins of conclusions based on the fact that people didn't care about me, and therefore I must not be worth caring for.

My point of view created my reality, and informed how I engaged with the world and participated in every relationship. I felt isolated and alone. The world was unreliable. Nothing and no one could be trusted to care for me, including me. My conclusions did not allow me to see anything different that did not match what I fundamentally believed to be true, and I diligently gathered evidence for the truth and proof of my conclusions everywhere in every relationship.

I suffered inside these coffins of conclusion, rejecting all other possibilities, until just a few years ago. What changed?

The Disillusionment of A Reality of Lies

Again, I will thank Gary Douglas and the tools of Access Consciousness® for contributing to the dynamic difference my life is today. In 2010, I attended Level 2 and 3 classes with Gary Douglas in San Francisco and he called me a liar for four days. I was stunned and confused. It was confronting to say the least. I could not comprehend why he maintained I was lying when I responded to every question he asked me with what I believed to be complete truth. What was he talking about? Finally on the fourth day of class, feeling quite exasperated and discouraged, one last question occurred to me. I asked Gary this. "What is it going to take to know when I'm lying to myself?" He responded with one word, "Vulnerability."

I had no idea what he meant by that response. Vulnerability was dangerous. It was the very thing I had been defending against all my life. I thought vulnerability left me exposed to pain, oppression and victimization, and I had spent a life-time carefully constructing a fortress of protection to ensure that never happened. Little did I realize that the very fortress I thought was protecting me from the threat of harm was the very same construct of judgment I used to invoke and per-petuate the trauma of separation from being.

I left those classes in San Francisco with a newfound determi-nation to experiment with vulnerability as a way of research-ing possibility. It turns out the vulnerability I so vehemently avoided was the healing elixir that would guide me home.

The Five Elements of Intimacy

As a pioneer of consciousness, I am willing to put on my lab coat and enter the laboratory called life to do whatever inves-tigation is required in discovering what else is possible. For the last five years, I have been exploring the five elements of intimacy as presented by Access Consciousness®. My deliberate attention in cultivating these five elements has awakened an intimacy of being that I never before imagined possible. Healing the primary trauma and separation from being has transpired quite naturally through my exploration, and judgment as a vital strategy for separation and protec-tion has ceased to be of any relevance or value.

The five elements of intimacy are honor, trust, allowance, vulnerability and gratitude.

Honor

When functioning from judgment, all possibility of honoring anyone or anything is excluded. I unceremoniously dismissed being when I adopted the evaluative strategy of judgment that consensus reality so desperately depends upon. The more I began seeing through the "lie glasses" of the judgment my parents impelled on me, the more performance-based behavior emerged shaped by their rewarding approval and withholding disapproval. Being was dismissed and cast aside as inconsequential.

In cultivating the elements of intimacy, I had to go looking for the kindness that had all but been eliminated from my reality via judgment. In support of my choice to relinquish any dependency on judgment, I repeatedly asked this question as a request for something greater. "What energy, space and consciousness of infinite kindness can I be and receive right now with total ease?" I had to summon the energy of honor. To honor is to be kind, to treat with regard and receive being irrespective of conditionally appropriate behavior. I found honor, and dissolved the barriers to communion with being, when I finally removed the "lie glasses" of judgment I mistakenly thought would protect me.

Trust

When I operated from the point of view that I needed to control my external environment to ensure I was safe from anything I considered a threat, I believed trust to be a means of preventing pain. I would evaluate others to determine whether I believed they were more or less likely to do what I wanted them to do. I decided to trust them if I concluded they were more likely to do what I expected of them. But, trust in this way could only provide a false sense of security. My decision to trust them based on judgment based evaluations and conclusions cut me off from any awareness of all they were capable of being, doing and choosing. I was blind-sided by this version of trust more times than I can count.

Now, I now trust others to be, do and choose whatever they are going to be, do and choose. I trust them implicitly to know what is true for them, and make no effort to control what they choose. I trust what I know implicitly, and know that I am not at the effect of anyone else's choice. This unconditional trust allows me to receive everything that arises in life with greater ease, and simply choose. And, choice creates. Remember?

Allowance

Judgment scorns allowance. Everything in my life was subject to the discriminating weapon of judgment, which I wielded uncompromisingly. There was no room for error, and I took pride in my capacity to preemptively judge all I was doing wrong according to consensus reality. I arrogantly informed anyone eager to judge me that they need not bother with the effort of it because I would administer any punishing judgment in a far more wrathful way than they likely ever would. True story.

Through practicing allowance, I began to realize that everything is just an interesting point of view. The judgments I had fortified my life with were not as factually real as I thought. I recognized that judgment is completely subjective, and its destructive impact on my life could only endure to the degree I solidified it as real and relevant as an effective strategy for functioning.

I created dynamic shifts in my life when I discovered that being in allowance is a lubricant of change. It acts as an antidote to judgment dissolving its paralyzing effects, and opens the doorways of possibility that judgment eliminates. Choosing into the space of allowance revealed a reality beyond the construct of good and bad, right and wrong.

Allowance is a gateway to receiving. As I live in greater allowance, I create more ease and intimacy of being with everyone and everything. That ease is the byproduct of an absence of wrongness, or even rightness, when living in allowance. When judgment is absent, receiving is present, and I effortlessly enjoy the limitlessness of functioning as an infinite being.

Vulnerability

I am a recovering control freak of magnitude. Throughout my life, I struggled to control just about everything in my reality in order to prevent the experiences I wanted to avoid, so I would never have to feel what I feared too painful to feel. I controlled things in an attempt to escape everything I decided was threatening. That control was an absolute refusal of receiving, and the effort required to get what I blocked from receiving was exhausting. Accomplishing anything seemed increasingly difficult, and living felt arduous.

Vulnerability is only possible in the absence of control. It is being without barriers to anyone or anything. It is living in question rather than always needing an answer, and concluding before you choose.

Functioning as an infinite being, and choosing new possibilities beyond consensus reality requires vulnerability. As I tenaciously chose greater vulnerability by giving up any necessity for control, I discovered something quite unexpected about being vulnerable. It is the source of an inherent potency far greater than any degree of power derived from judgment, and all my rigorous efforts to control, could have ever been. Perhaps consensus reality would prefer that game changing revelation be kept a secret?

The intensity of vulnerability is often interpreted as scared or afraid. When I misidentified it in this way, I was unable to move beyond the refuge of the familiar into the awkward unknown of the possible. Sustained transformative change requires vulnerability. Dissolving all barriers to communion with being and the willingness to receive everything without judgment allowed me to know and live the potency of vulnerability.

Gratitude

Gratitude is not accessible in the presence of judgment. I had been taught by my parents to be thankful for things like gifts and all the essential provisions of a secure life that were provided for me. They often told me that many people around the world lived with much less, and I should be grateful. Yet with the presence of judgment so prevalent, that version of thankfulness always felt compulsory and full of effort. The energy of gratitude I discovered while exploring the five elements of intimacy is something altogether different.

Gratitude, I noticed, appeared quite naturally when I stopped choosing against, and separating from, being via judgment. Joy-filled gratitude is innate to being. Deliberately cultivating the five elements of intimacy dissolved barriers to communion with being, and I became aware of the contribution everything is to my life and the contribution intimacy of being is to everyone and everything. I perceive the abundant vitality of energy continually gifted by a magnanimous universe, and have gratitude for all that is expanding into infinite possibility. It's so very delicious!

Healing Through Intimacy of Being

For me, healing is a day-by-day practice of choosing intimacy of being rather than the separation of judgment. Intimacy of being is where I trust what I know with an absence of doubt. Living this way has gifted me the awareness that nothing is wrong and nothing is missing, and being is not a judgeable offense. Without the judgment that created separation from being, nothing is absent and communion with all things is present. I became aware that any pain or harm I had so furiously labored to avoid and prevent isn't even real. What I had concluded as harm cannot even occur, except by choice through separation from being and dismissing awareness.

The barriers I maintained as a way to separate and isolate began to dissolve in a way that was quite natural. They simply stopped being useful as I recognized I did not need them. They just went away.

Healing through intimacy of being revealed that the pain I had believed was caused by so many others in my life was a lie. The primary trauma of abandoning being was actually the only pain I had ever felt though I spent a lifetime blaming others as its cause. I realized no harm could come to me unless I separated from being and awareness first. The conclusion that control would secure safety was exposed as a lie, and I chose vulnerability in its place. As I broke the spell of each coffin of conclusion, the pain I had attributed to everything other than choice began to release. The peace, ease and joy of being became more real than any of the stories I had maintained as supportive evidence for the need and necessity of separation.

In this space of communion is healing. Judgment having lost its usefulness becomes obsolete.

Being Home

Every day I choose living intimately in communion with being, which allows me to receive everyone and everything. When someone delivers judgment or unkindness, it does not register as relevant to me anymore. I recognize it simply as information about how they are functioning. It reveals to me everywhere they have not yet let go of the lies they imprison being with, and so remain compelled to maintain a dependence on judgment as power and protection. Before I embarked on my journey home to being, I resided in that prison too. The five elements of intimacy were each keys that allowed me to confront the lies that imprisoned me and allowed me to live free, finally home in the intimacy of being.

About the Author

TAMARA YOUNKER

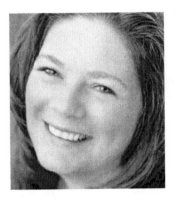

Tamara Younker is a Certified Facilitator, Coach, Mediator, Speaker and pioneer of consciousness who has been researching the energetics of relating for 13 years. She has an expertise in guiding clients to cultivate Intimacy of Being where they function from a powerful and aware presence that allows them to live more creatively in the world and less at the effect of it.

It's Tamara's desire to contribute to the emergence of a new paradigm for interpersonal relating, one that arises from allowance and choice rather than judgment and control. She facilitates Access Consciousness Core Classes internationally, as well as, her own specialty classes on Intimacy. Her joy is inviting others to give up their current dependence on judgment as a valuable strategy for separation and protection, so the intimacy of Oneness with all things becomes a natural way of living for all.

Chapter 5

How to Access Your Inner Physician and Heal Your Body

Dr. Kim D'Eramo

"Is it serious?" she asked. Molly sat in the flimsy hospital gown, barely covered from her thighs up and feeling completely exposed otherwise.

"Well, we're really not sure. It depends. Sometimes. It's typically life-long...but I have some medications we'll try that should help with the symptoms." Her doctor's stumbled words betrayed his confident demeanor, but he quickly recomposed himself as he took out his prescription pad and patted the table in an attempt to reassure her.

There had been little eye-contact during the appointment and Molly felt like he hadn't really seen her. She didn't like what she was hearing, but she'd been suffering with body aches, muscle spasms, joint pain, and sleepless nights for months without a solution. Somehow, having a real diagnosis felt reassuring, so she accepted her fate. The previous doctors had made her feel like this was all in her head.

"I have fi-bro-my-alg-ia," she later confidently told her sister. *That's what's been going on all this time. I knew there was a problem."*

"Fibro-what?" was the reply.

This story describes the scene in millions of doctors' offices today. People with low energy, weight gain, pain, anxiety, depression...being given a strange diagnosis and then being treated with one of the latest medications advertised and promoted by the drug companies. All in a 15-minute doctor visit.

More than half of adults today have been diagnosed with a chronic illness. Twenty-five percent of all adults have more than one chronic illness, and these numbers are climbing. Soon there will be more sick people in our country than healthy people. Most have been given more than one pharmaceutical medication as the solution to treat their symptoms. Few of them are expected to become free from disease.

Is this the best we can do?

No wonder so many people feel hopeless to heal, despite their natural desire to have vitality and wellbeing.

As an Emergency Medicine doctor, I see these patients turning to the medical system for help. They're looking to be vibrant and whole, but will settle for medications to get them out of pain. No one is letting them know there are other options. Few doctors have gone to the trouble to research what can be done to actually help the body heal. Certainly there isn't time in our current system for doctors to do much more than a quick fix, a band-aid; but couldn't we at least inform patients about those who can?

Today's healthcare workers are excellent at keeping you alive and delaying death, but very poor at helping you be truly healthy and well.

What is health and wellness, anyway?

The truth is, doctors learn nothing about health in medical school. The term "healthcare" system is a misnomer. What we learn about in medical training is disease. We have created a disease-care system. We're very, very good at managing disease...but for patients who want wellbeing and vitality, it doesn't really matter.

I had the fortune of training as an osteopathic physician, which means that during medical school, I did learn about how the body heals. I learned that the mind and body are one, and that the body has the ability to heal itself, and I've seen this MindBody connection and self-healing mechanism do amazing and miraculous things...like reverse chronic illness for good. I know the immense power of the body, so when patients tell me "my doctor said my illness is life-long and nothing can be done," I know that just isn't true.

If the body has the ability to heal itself, why are so many people suffering? The problem comes from our perspective. Einstein said that a problem cannot be solved at the same level at which it was created. What this means relative to your health is, you can't "fix" the problem. You can only create the circumstances in which the problem doesn't exist. That's why going to the conventional doctor will typically not lead you to a solution.

How can we support the body in being free from illness? Stop focusing on the problem, and *focus on the solution*.

Whenever I approach a patient, I immediately begin looking for the root cause for their illness. I know the body has the ability to be vibrantly healthy, so something is keeping it from doing that. Either the body is not getting what it needs, or it's getting too much of something it does not need. This can be on a physical, mental, or emotional level. (Some practitioners talk about the spiritual level of health, but to me, everything is spirit, and we can't really separate that.)

Physical root causes can be related to nutrition. Not enough creates a nutritional deficiency, and too much creates toxicity. Physical causes can also be movement related. Not enough exercise prevents the body from releasing tensions and strains, or staying flexible and limber so it can realign itself. Too much movement creates injury or wear on the body. These are generalizations, but physical root causes, as simple as they are, are still typically not addressed by conventional doctors.

Mental and emotional root causes of illness are much more pervasive and are present with virtually every chronic illness I've seen. This is where the Mind-Body connection comes into play. Every thought you have creates chemical reactions that affect everything in your body. The tension in your muscles, your metabolism and weight, your ability to digest food well, and even how fast you age are all primarily determined not by your age or genetic code, but by your level of thought.

There was a study done that reversed aging in an elderly nursing home population. When the group of 80-something year old patients were brought to a camp that reflected a much earlier era —a time when they would have been 18 years old- they experienced profound changes in their health. Not only did they feel better —pain decreased, sleep improved, and energy levels were higher, but they also became physically younger. Their heart rate and blood pressure improved, cholesterol levels decreased, and immune markers went up. The 18-year old mindset created substantial and significant health changes in their body.

These folks were able to do things they weren't previously able to do like carry their own heavy baggage, and run without pain. It was a miracle! Or was it? If you hold the perspective that the aging process is inevitable, and disease can only be treated with medications, than this would seem like a miracle. If, however, you understand the power of thought and mindset on the physical body, then this makes perfect scientific sense.

What about our emotions? Emotions play a very large role in our health, and stuck emotions are the largest blocks to healing. Think about it, have you ever had a paper cut? It may be super painful, but you know why you got it, you know it will heal fast, and you know it's no big deal. Maybe you're annoyed for a few moments, but you let it go, and the cut heals. Now think about chronic pain: you don't know why it's happening, you don't know when it will come or go, and you don't know if it could be something serious. It freaks you out and you carry it continuously. All patients I've seen with chronic pain have frustration and annoyance at best, and fear and powerlessness at worst that are associated with their symptoms. When I've helped them release the emotions, the pain resolves, sometimes instantly!

The new model of medicine I propose takes into account the mental and emotional affects on our health. When we focus only on the physical symptoms, we're looking just at the tip of the iceberg. We can treat with medications all day long, (and we do!) but until we look at what's causing this physical disturbance on the mental and emotional levels, the patient will continue to require medications or other treatment. Using supplements, therapy or diet to manage symptoms is the same. If your body's not reversing the illness, it's because you are only managing the symptoms. You're dealing with the tip of the iceberg and not eliminating the root causes.

When we address root causes, there is no more disease. When we address the root causes, the body manages the rest. This takes the pressure off the healer to micromanage all of the symptoms. When we remember that the body has it handled, we can give the body what it needs and leave the rest up to the body's inner healer.

We all have an inner healer. This is your personal guru and is more powerful and wise than any doctor. The key is listening and tuning in for information.

Our current healthcare system is disempowering. Patients are disempowered because they have to rely on the doctor to tell them what's going on in their body and what they should do. Doctors are disempowered because they're educated primarily by the pharmaceutical industry, and not tuning into their own intuition and inner wisdom to explore possibilities and solutions. When we tune in and listen to our inner healer, there are always answers that lead to solutions. The answers may be to take action and visit a doctor or other practitioner, or to take medication or other remedies, but these will come from a sense of certainty and security, instead of powerlessness and disconnection.

How do we listen to our inner healer for guidance and solutions?

This is the true art of medicine that has been increasingly overlooked in the past decades. When I see patients (typically over Skype since I now consult with clients all over the world) I guide them through this process of inner knowing and we discover the answers together. We then clear whatever is holding them back from expressing complete health and vibrance. The results are amazing.

In this chapter, I'm going to guide you through this process to use for yourself. We all have the ability to get this kind of information from our body's inner wisdom. You may need to practice often, and you may want to seek support with this process.

Here's what your MindBody is really capable of that will dramatically diminish the drug companies' business:

You're not broken.

Although it seems like you're a solid, static being, separate from everything else, the truth is: *you are made of energy.* Your body is in constant motion, is constantly changing, and is connected to everything else.

As a separate, solid, static being it makes sense to think that when there's a problem in your system you need something outside of you to fix it. Medications introduce new chemical reactions to alter what's happening and fix the problem. In this line of thinking, if you have "bad genes," that's unlucky and there's not much you can do about it. However, the true problem is not at the level of your genes or the chemical reactions in your body. The real problem is the *"energy blueprint"* that put that chemistry into motion.

When we realize that we're not solid, we're not separate, and we're not static, the whole game changes. As energy, our bodies are in constant flux, are intimately connected with everything around us, AND are powerfully influenced by our mind and emotions. It's like your cells are constantly listening to the blueprint set up by your mindset.

Your mind is constantly communicating with your body, and it has the ability to affect and influence everything going on in your health and your life. Your mind impacts energy – your energy, and the energy around you. You are more powerful than you can imagine. Let's use this power to transform your health.

First, Get In Your Body

You must bring your awareness and attention into your body before you can use your mind to create what you want or enhance your health. The first step to intentionally using the power of your mind is to *get present*. Typically, people spend time with their awareness focused outside the body and outside the present moment. You could be focusing on social media, email or text messages, with none of your awareness inside your body. You could also be engaged in a conversation with little of your attention present to experience it.

You could even be exercising outside of your body! If you're on a treadmill reading a book or watching TV, with little if any of your attention on what's going on in your body, you're not really present. Interestingly, this significantly limits the benefits of exercise and it will take you far longer to achieve results.

As soon as you bring your awareness into your body by feeling your physical body, your energy comes back in and you can begin to use it to create health.

Next, Take Back Your Power

You have the power to choose the health and the life you love. You lose this power, however, consciously or unconsciously, when you adopt beliefs and perspectives that limit you. Your power to heal and to choose your life gets dissipated when you're caught up with old stories, limited beliefs, or ideas you've adopted about yourself and about life that aren't really true. In so doing, your energy is fragmented and not harnessed into the areas that serve you most.

Think of your thoughts like records playing in your mind. You've assigned part of your energy system to play these records with thoughts, ideas, and beliefs. These records inform your system. If your records are saying: *"Life is difficult,"* your brain activity limits itself to seeing difficulty. It changes the information coming you're your mind, so you only see difficult choices, difficult situations, and difficult people.

These records can serve you. If you've assigned part of your energy to play a record to the tune of: *"Life is easy and The Universe is on my side,"* then your brain activity is consistent with that: You see opportunities right in front of you. You see the best in other people and enjoy them, and your body receives messages that enhance your performance and mental clarity. Things, thus, are easy.

There are four ways your body can lose energy with these records playing in your mind: *Past, Future, I, and Other.* I learned this from Richard Moss, who was one of my spiritual teachers.

When your energy and awareness is in the past, you have records playing about old stories, things that happened to you, things you should have done differently, how someone wronged you, or how things didn't go the way you wanted them to. When your energy is focused in the past, this brings up *anger, sadness, resentment, and grief.*

You can also scatter part of your energy and awareness in the future. When the records playing in your mind are about what might happen, how you might not get what you need, or how you might lose something that you have...you are putting your energy and attention in the future. When this occurs, there is *fear, anxiety and overwhelm.* Typically, people have tendencies toward one area or the other.

The best way to quickly bring your energy and attention back where it can serve you is to bring your attention into your body. The body only lives in the present moment. It can never live in the past or live in the future. (If this doesn't make sense, try.) When you feel your body, this immediately unhooks your energy from past and future, and brings it into the "Now," where everything happens.

The body only lives in the present moment.

The other ways we lose energy from our body is when it's caught up in "Other" or "I," or self-identity. When you are blaming others, wondering what your mother would say, or upset about something someone said, your mind records are playing tunes about "Other." You are investing energy in people outside of yourself.

What about "I?" If the records in your head are playing thoughts about what it means to be a man/woman, a wife/husband, or the fact that you're a doctor, a lawyer, a 50-year old person, a "vegan," or a "Democrat," part of your energy is caught up in self-identification and can hold you back from healing. How you identify yourself affects your body and your experiences in life.

To bring your energy out of "Other" or "I," simply bring your awareness and attention into your body. Be present not to who you *think* you are, (which is totally based on ideas, thoughts, and beliefs) but who you ARE. There's a huge difference. Who you think you are is about the definitions you've developed or others have given you about yourself. It's about information and ideas. It will always be limited. Who you *really* are is about awareness and truth. Your body will give you truth. You must, however, be present to receive it.

Change Your State

Now that you have retrieved your energy and gathered it into your body, you can use it to heal. Relaxation is the most important part of healing. When your muscles relax, you are more connected with the world around you, with energy and what's going on around you, and with The Universe and its wisdom.

Breathing slowly and deeply allows your body to relax and keeps your awareness anchored in your body, so you use it to heal. Breathing this way also balances your nervous system. It turns off the "fight or flight" response that generates harmful chemicals that cause disease, and ignites the "relaxation response" that restores balance, heath, and wellbeing.

Calm Your Brain

Once you've slowed your breathing, and brought it deeper into your body, your brain activity slows down. You come out of the "high beta" frequency of analysis, calculation, and fast-paced thoughts, and into a slower "low-beta" or "alpha" state that allows your brain to process new information, perceive opportunities, think creatively and function at peak performance. In this slower brain wave state your brain is able to accept affirming beliefs, ideas and wisdom, such as: *"I am powerful, healthy, and strong."* Basically, this enables you to update those old records playing in the back of your mind to life-enhancing background music that keeps you vibrant and healthy.

A great way to ground this slower brain wave state is to bring your attention deeper into your body. When your awareness is in your head, this increases brain processing and speeds things up in a way that does not benefit you.

It may seem that you think with your head, but as you will soon see, you "think" with your whole body. Your mind goes beyond the boundaries of your physical form.

Bringing your attention deeper into your body allows your brain to enter a more balanced level of activity, and allows you to access your inner wisdom and inner healer.

Create Your Future

Your brain does not know the difference between the real and the imagined. So when you imagine being vibrant, healthy, joyful and fit, you activate the same regions of your brain as when you are experiencing these states. That allows you to inform your brain of where you're going and what you want to experience. It's like setting the destination on your GPS. Your mind will lead you to the destination you plug in. Setting your intention and visualizing it to activate brain activity is how you plug in your coordinates for where you want to go.

Your mind, communicates in images. When you imagine yourself running on the beach, holding your loved ones, or cheering with joy, it registers this on every level of your being. This change in brain activity generates the hormones, neurochemicals and immune components that create vibrant health and create the result you envision.

You can create any kind of intention you want and you don't have to know how you're going to bring it about. Your mind is infinitely creative and will guide you in the right direction. Investing in this process is one of the smartest ways you can use your energy, and can save you years of wasted time and effort.

I created a video for you that takes you through the process of connecting with your inner healer.

You can access it for free at:

DrKimD.com/EnergyofHealing

Accessing Your Inner Physician Exercise:

1. Get present in your body. Feel your feet on the floor. Feel your bum on the seat. Relax your shoulders away from your ears. Bring all of your awareness into your body.

2. Take deep breaths as your belly balloons out, then exhale as your belly comes back in. Slow and deepen your breathing as you breathe several breaths like this.

3. Pull your awareness from your head down into your body. Start by imagining that there's a magnet inside your head that gathers all of your energy into your head. Past, future, focus on work or others in your life releases, and you simply bring all parts of you into your head.

4. Place an imaginary second magnet in your chest, and imagine this magnet pulling your energy and attention into your body around your heart.

5. Now place a third magnet down at your core. This magnet is located just below the belly button in your pelvis. See if you can bring all of your attention and energy here. Have this magnet pull your energy all the way down to your pelvis.

6. Imagine being at your ideal state of health. This might be you enjoying exercise or activities you could only do when you're healthy. It might be you celebrating with friends and enjoying delicious foods that you otherwise aren't able to

enjoy, or you waking up refreshed and smiling as you go about your morning routine.

The mind communicates in symbols and images, so you want to see images that match your ideal state of health. Just focus your mind on these images.

7. Ask your body: *"What would it take for me to live in this state now?"* Then feel the energy that comes up in your body. There may be an idea, a feeling, a color, an image, a word, or a sound. Whatever comes up, bring your awareness onto this energy.

This may be difficult at first, if you are not used to listening to your body and feeling your own energy. Just trust whatever comes up.

8. Clear what's in the way of you living in this state of health. State to your body: *"Everything that's in the way of this, I delete, un-create, and destroy."* Feel into the energy that's in the way. Feel your choice to let go of all that has been in the way. Is there resistance to doing this?

(If there is resistance to releasing the old energy, like not believing it could be that simple or a feeling that it's not really going anywhere, simply state: *"All the disbelief, doubt and fear that's holding back, I delete, uncreate and destroy now."* Do this until you feel a sense of freedom and ease, like you know the energy of well being is available to you and it's ok.)

9. Incorporate this energy of healing into your body. See the

energy of healing move into your physical body and restore your health. Feel it incorporate into every cell, informing a new level of energy, vitality, and wellbeing.

10. Finish with a few deep, slow breaths to integrate this energy and celebrate your new life.

Please be sure to watch the more extended version of this MindBody tool at: DrKimD.com/EnergyofHealing.

I look forward to supporting you as together we create a world free from chronic illness.

Blessings for your health!

About the Author
DR. KIM D'ERAMO

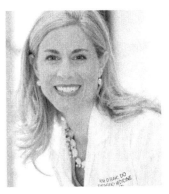

Dr. Kim D'Eramo is a physician, speaker, bestselling author of The MindBody Tool Kit, and founder of The American Institution of MindBody Medicine. She is board-certified in Emergency Medicine, and trained at Emory University's Grady Hospital in Atlanta. She attended medical school at University of New England College of Osteopathic Medicine, where she also completed fellowship training in Osteopathic Medicine, Gross Anatomy and Neuroanatomy.

Dr. D'Eramo healed herself from a chronic illness doctors told her would be life-long and require medications indefinitely. She now teaches internationally, to empower patients with tools that immediately reverse symptoms and activate the body's healing capacity. Dr. D'Eramohas researched for decades the pathways through which the body heals itself, and has formulated this into tools that can be used any time to repattern the brain, send new messages to the body, and restore ideal health physically, emotionally and mentally.

Dr. D'Eramo currently sees clients online for transformational healing. She conducts online group training programs, and speaks nationally to doctors, and the general public for training in MindBody Medicine. Dr. Kim has appeared multiple times on local and national television as well as multiple media publications. Receive your free MindBody tools today at: DrKimD.com.

Chapter 6

Changing What
You Think You Cannot
Change

By Katherine McIntosh

Can you imagine what it would be like if you knew that you could change any ailment in your body and life?

Have you ever met someone who is still talking about something that happened to them over 30 years ago and they are bitter, enraged, and still trying to let go of the experience as if someone else was responsible for the pain they haven't yet let go of?

I remember being on the big island of Hawaii, lush tropical land, the sound of the ocean waves hitting the walls of volcanic rock, the wind, the breeze, the joy...the dance. I had landed on The Big Island for a Shamanic Retreat. I entered the room and sat down in a circle that went from youngest to eldest. It was a sign of respect for Shamanic Circles to honor the wisdom of our elders. We were initiating our circle by sharing what we were here to let go of and what we were there to initiate and activate in every area of our life. There was an elderly man, one of the last of the group to share his story. I remember him pointing to me, the third youngest of 25 people and he said he wished he had known when he was my age that he could let go of the pain, rage, and bitterness he was still hanging onto from his parents who were now on the other side. His trembling voice eked out the pain in words as he said: "I still haven't made peace with something that happened to me 50+ years ago and I am dying because of it."

He was dying from a story that was deep in his bones as a history that was more real than the possibility of the present moment. It was sad and I knew there had to be a different way of living.

Dying to live was not the path I was willing to walk and in that moment I demanded that I would not carry any pain and resentment from my childhood. I would change my story.

Fast forward to over a decade and I have done exactly that. I have decided that the present moment offers a way greater way of living than ranting about any past experience even if it was filled with pain, abuse, neglect, and any other form of self defeat that comes from being a kid in a family that doesn't understand you.

I have become known in the healing and entrepreneurial industry as someone willing to defy the odds and use a little bit of magic to create a different possibility. When you are willing to acknowledge that magic is our birthright, as opposed to pain, then you encounter examples of magic defying possibilities to help you align with the reality that you know is true.

I was recently at a weekend mastermind with 6- and 7-figure Conscious Business owners and I started a conversation with a stunning blonde from Europe. She embodied the definition of external and internal beauty. She was 5'10" tall, with long blonde perfectly highlighted hair, porcelain skin, amazing sense of fashion, great humor, and her personality shined through her being. I remember seeing her and thinking what it would be like to be her..... to have that level of perfection, a body that I would have at one time in my life done absolutely anything to have. At one point, I almost died trying to have that perfect body.

I was curious and wanted to know what it would be like to be in her skin. I wondered so many different things including her story and what she had done in her life to be sitting amongst a room full of highly successful entrepreneurs. In a moment of connection, I started to ask her questions about her and her life.

Here was this beautiful blonde that had a striking personality to match her striking beauty and she began describing her experience of her once crippled, bed-ridden body.

She was a dancer and creative genius at heart. At the age of 15, she had a snowboard accident that left her paralyzed from the waist down. She shattered her back and spine in multiple places leaving her to lay still in bed as if she was in a coma. Paralyzed and in bed for five straight months, the doctors told her she would never move, dance, play, ski, snowboard, and move her body again. She was furious, depressed, upset, and utterly confused. Doctors told her that she would never be able to walk or play or move again.

I was shocked to hear her story, her experience, and her pain that pierced through her body and spirit. There were no remaining physical or emotional scars, except for the ones I could perceive that still remained in the bones of her pelvis and hips.

She was standing upright, glowing inside and out, and I was stunned to hear of the pain that once crippled her body and spirit. No one would ever know by looking at her.

Fascinated, I asked her: "How did you heal?"

Her response was: "By believing that something else was possible". She said that when the doctor's told her she couldn't move, her entire body trembled with anger and rage. She couldn't buy their diagnosis as true. She had been connected to her body her whole life and she said there was no way she could buy that the disconnect from her accident was a permanent prognosis she had to swallow as if she was being force fed the wrong dose of medicine.

She decided not to swallow the wrong pill and went on a journey to discover what else is possible.

She found healing by connecting with the right people.... people who were willing to defy the impossible. By talking to her nerve endings, getting physical support, and hands-on healing from a particular alternative healer, she did the impossible. She healed her crippled body and reconnected the severed nerves that were causing her to be paralyzed.

My response was: "Of course you did" and I began to share my own knowledge of the body and how that very knowledge defies the wisdom that we are taught from this reality's perspective.

We are told that if you are sick, you go to a doctor. You get medicine for a cold, aspirin for a headache, a cast for a broken bone, chemo for cancer, surgery for removable tumors, pills for ADD, ADHD, erectile disfunction, rheumatoid arthritis, etc. The list goes on and on and on, but the essential message we are taught to buy is that someone else has the answer for what's wrong with you.

I have a different version of that as a reality.

There is nothing wrong with you!

You are a genius. You are magic. You don't need fixing.

You need to be shown that the genius inside of you is waiting to be

acknowledged, played with, and nurtured. And if something is challenging in your body or life, then you just need the necessary support to get the healing and support you need.

So as this woman told her story, it was validation, and proof of the magic we and our bodies are capable of....we just need to be shown the way.

Within nine months she was standing, walking, and moving her pelvis. Granted, her body still had a long way to go to find herself somewhat upright. By the time she was able to stand, she still looked like a cripple: her body still a failed contortion from her once erect, posture-perfect dancing frame.

How does that happen? How does one go from permanently paralyzed for the rest of her life, to full, healed, vibrant and dancing again? How does one heal stage 4 cancer with alternative modes of healing? How does one defy the odds and change reality?

There is no logical explanation that can describe this. Instead, I believe there is a force far greater than any of us. I believe this very force is inside each of us as a seed, waiting for the right amount of water and sunshine to blossom into a fully grown flower. Call it God, Allah, Buddha, spirit, Jesus..... Call it whatever you want, but when odds are completely defied, then there is a force far greater than anything we can ever imagine: I call it MAGIC!

It is the body and mind's natural ability to heal itself. How does that happen?

I believe that it boils down to one thing: believing that you can. Never giving up, never giving in, never stopping, and always finding your way to the space of possibility despite the odds stacked against you.

What if true healing wasn't what you thought?

What if it required fierce determination and a giant dose of magic?

How do you cognitively explain that?

From my perspective, true healing is kind of like going on an adventure where you may have an end in sight, but you don't exactly know what the journey will bring. When I was 23, I spent six weeks backpacking through all of South America. I wanted to see as many sites and mountains, and lands, and ruins, and bodies of water, and different people, and cities that I could possibly do in those six weeks. I didn't have much of a plan except to follow the energy. That one experience paved much of how I created my life as an adventure of possibility instead of a calculated plan where I needed to stick to a schedule.

I suck at plans and if you've ever traveled in South America, or any other country that prides itself on taking it's time and going with the flow, then you know there is NO PLAN. A plan is a calculated set of actions that seldom take into account a hail storm, or a tsunami, or any other distraction that causes you to take a completely different course of action.

I look at healing anything, the body, mind, spirit, a broken heart, a broken leg, or a shattered marriage as an unplanned journey that must follow guidance, intuition, and an inner knowing that you cannot totally plan for.

This reality teaches you that in order to heal something you have to have the answer to solve the thing you think is the problem. If you and your body are always changing, then doesn't that also mean that the cure changes too?

True healing is your body's natural state. The body is designed to regenerate itself in its entirety every seven years. It is astounding what the body is capable of. The trick is that we have to allow it to DO it's genius. If we get in the way because we think we have a better plan than nature...well nature and the body will show you an entirely different truth.

But you have to listen.

And if you don't, that's when the pain, or disease, or fatigue, or exhaustion, or suffering take place.

Are you in charge of your body or is your body in charge of you? Have you ever tried to lose weight and your body started to gain weight instead? Is that because you had control of your body, or because your body had control of you? Control is about trying to force an outcome. And in my experience, forcing an outcome never allows for the spirit of a greater magic to contribute to a greater possibility.

I have a two and a half year-old son, and it is amazing to me how many bumps, bruises, scrapes, and bangs he will incur in a day, and within 24 hours, most of the evidence of the incident is gone. He doesn't have a point of view that when he flies through the air over the handle bars of his strider bike in super man form, thudding against an ice packed snow bank, that he shouldn't get back on his bike and keep going. He doesn't have a built in pathway in his brain that tries to inform him he needs to "sit it out for a minute". He just peels himself off the snow bank and gets back on his bike and keeps on riding.

When he falls hard, I usually ask him if he hurt the cement or the floor and he'll get up, get a strange look on his face and walk away. He is tough AND he doesn't have a point of view that pain is wrong. He is programmed to trust the resilience of his body and the magic of the body's natural capacity to heal itself.

He inspires me and shows me magic with his body every day...not just in healing, but he is close to defying nature as a 2.5 year-old that is fierce, fearless, and full of energy that trusts MAGIC is a part of his very existence.

Our bodies come in with the natural ability to heal anything and when we don't have a point of view about that healing (or the pain or the disease)...how long it will take to change, how fast, how much, then the body can regenerate itself quickly, like magic.

I am aware that 10,000 cells die every second while 10,000 new cells are being born every second. That means our bodies regenerate themselves in their entirety every seven years....is that magic?

What do you know?

If you don't have a point of view about how your body can heal itself, what would your body do? What could it choose?

What if, you could ask your body a question? What if you could ask your being a question?

A question is designed to empower you to look at what you know. A question always brings up an energy that is information for you to look at. And it also engages the forces stronger than yourself to aid in the quest for what you are looking for. Something greater can happen.

If you are like most people you were taught at a young age to stop asking questions and to have all the answers. I believe that this structure eliminates you from discovering the power you have inside where you know better about yourself and your body and your life than anyone else.

True healing isn't about getting rid of something. True healing is about using everything as information to create a greater possibility. True healing is about acknowledging that who you are as a being, right now, is enough.

You are more than enough.

I was born and raised Irish Catholic. My parents were rather traditional. If something was broken, it got fixed by a doctor, a psychologist, a mechanic, or something else.

I was born a psychic/intuitive with parents who couldn't ever imagine their child knew something outside of the norms of what the bible dictated. I was a bit out of place in my family of origin. Instead of knowing that I was different, I always thought something was wrong with me.

The psychologist's office was an all too familiar place where judgment and wrongness were the solid confines of my teenage confusion, only more reason to rebel against my parents and solidify even further the deep groove of distance I felt between me and the rest of the world, especially my family.

You see, no one told me I had a gift. I just thought there was something wrong with me, so I went on what felt like a never ending (expensive) quest to discover what it would take to make the madness and pain inside of me stop.

I spent 20 years of self discovery, studying to get my master's degree in Somatic Psychology, reading, and learning about every modality you could possibly think of and almost nothing changed the internal turmoil until one day in my late 20s, on the verge of falling apart, sick and withering to the bone, desperate to change my "disease", I walked into a woman's office. She put her hands on my sacrum and lower belly and spent 30 minutes asking me and my body questions.

An hour later, I walked out of her office with a sense of relief and a deep inner knowing I had changed what doctors, therapists (and myself) had spent my entire life thinking I couldn't change. Prior to that session, I had spent the previous six months in and out of doctor's offices, blood tests, MRIs, CAT scans, pee tests and everything else you could think of. No one could figure out what was "wrong" with me.

I had given the power over to everyone else to figure out what was wrong with me, but that day...something had changed. It was the beginning of knowing that nothing was wrong with me. I wasn't broken. I didn't need fixing. I needed to know how truly brilliant and aware I was.

When I had that session, the woman wanted to know what I knew. She wanted to know what my body knew. She was inviting me to listen to what my body knew. Not from control, but from curiosity.

It was the first time anyone had ever bothered to truly be curious about what I knew. Here's what I discovered: I knew a lot more about me and my body than I thought. And as soon as I gave my body the attention it had been so desperately asking me to give it, it changed instantaneously.

It had been screaming at me for months, if not years. The volume of pain and intensity and discomfort kept getting louder and louder. I was trying to solve it by attempting to turn the volume down. But I wasn't willing to acknowledge that it wasn't about turning the volume down, it was about going underneath the surface to actually look at what the pain, intensity, and discomfort had been getting me to see. Once I was willing to actually acknowledge all of the energies I had been stuffing, everything changed.

It was a relief.

By looking underneath the surface, and actually talking and

listening to my body, I was able to heal not only my body, but my life.

Shortly after that experience I realized the power of asking questions. It was a power that had gifted me more than I knew was possible at the time.

That one-hour session changed the course of my life. All the doctors never bothered to ask me what was going on underneath the surface. They only wanted to address the symptom, but what I discovered underneath the surface was vital to creating the change that could be possible. And so, I went on a lifelong mission to discover the true capacities and mysteries and magic of healing.

True healing isn't about copying someone else's journey. True healing is about recognizing this is your journey: there is no one right answer, there are only questions, that lead to choices, that lead to possibilities. If we are trying to find the one solution that will solve everything, does it eliminate all the other solutions that could also work to create a different possibility?

Healing is about having choices. Seeing possibilities that don't yet exist and following your awareness. Healing is about allowing the body to do what it can do with the resources it has available. Healing is also about discovering you within the pain or disease so that magic can occur.

By being willing to acknowledge that my personal life was completely falling apart and I was miserable, the body pain, the cramping, the physical discomfort that was crippling me, disappeared almost overnight. I was finally listening.

When I discovered all of this information, I wanted to share it with everyone in my life whom I thought needed "healing". I wanted everyone to know what was possible...shout it to the rooftops. I wanted everyone to heal what they felt they couldn't. But what I discovered is that not many people were interested in changing what they already decided they couldn't.

When we are trying to find the one right solution that will solve the problem, we have to filter every answer through judgment.

Judgment is dense, it has a solidity to it. It does not create possibility. It stops the magic.

What if healing wasn't the issue, but the judgments we put on the issue that create the problem? It is our conclusion that stops the magic from changing everything almost instantaneously.

Healing, in my eyes, is always about creating space to new possibilities. It's the window of space that gives you a sense of peace in your universe. Healing is not about getting rid of something, so much as it is inviting the molecules of everything around you to organize to create more.

It's about inviting you to know what you know. When you hide yourself behind the should's and shouldn't's of what you think your story or your life should look like, you stop acknowledging that who you are is enough.

When you were born were you told that you were enough?

What if when you were born you were given a manual that showed you how magic you truly are? That your body is capable of sheer genius if you would actually listen to what it is trying to communicate.

In western medicine, we want to put a bandage on top of it, or a quick fix, or we want to swallow a magic pill to make it go away. But here's the thing, if you don't address what's causing it in the first place it will never go away.

What if the question was the answer? What then?

What I've discovered in my journey, is that no amount of therapy or judgment, or making myself wrong actually solved the problem. No amount of crucifying myself ever solved the problem.

It may sound crazy, but I've discovered true healing comes from being willing to look at the hard questions you don't want to look at.

When you're willing to abide by the saying: "ask and you shall receive", a different possibility becomes available. The question is not designed to make sure you come to an answer, the question is designed to give you an energetic download of the possibilities you never knew existed....which goes far beyond an answer. As soon as you acknowledge the energetic download, the information that was stuck has a chance to change.

There are no answers, only questions.

Once you come to a conclusion (also known as an answer)

the information stops...the change that's possible stops. Can you come to a conclusion with the weather?

NO.

I don't know about you, but I live in Colorado. The minute I think it's going to be a sunny day, the clouds roll in or the snow starts falling. Or vice versa. You can't come to a conclusion when it comes to the weather.

That's just like your bodies and your lives. The minute you conclude something is the answer or is concrete, it changes. Your bodies change, you change, your mind changes (especially if you're a woman), and your being changes.

True healing is about recognizing that everything is constantly in motion, changing, evolving, growing.

Have you ever had the experience of thinking you figured it out with your body, your relationships, your money? And the minute you've decided that it's figured out, it changes.

Throughout my career as an entrepreneur, I've watched myself say: "oh I figured out how to make money" and the minute I make that conclusion, the money slows down or stops.

What I've discovered in this journey is that healing is always in motion. Are you willing to allow it or do you need to stop it?

What if healing was being you no matter what?

What if you didn't have to make yourself wrong for what you think is wrong with you?

Is it ever light to hand over the authority of your body to someone else to tell you what you NEED to do?

When you were growing up as a teenager, did you like following your parents advice?

No!

I don't know about you, but I rebelled against every advice my parents tried to give me.

I couldn't follow any advice they offered, even if it was for my own good. I had to rebel. When you give your body over to an authority outside of yourself, your body rebels like a pissed off teenager. Your body has information inside that is screaming at you to pay attention. Instead of giving it a pill, freaking out, going immediately to the doctor, ask a question. See what you know and then go from there.

It's not that western medicine doesn't serve. It does. I've been to several doctors over the years that actually helped my own healing. The difference is that I didn't take what they said as true, I filtered their diagnosis through my own knowing. I listened and asked my body to show me what it needed, what was true for me, and what I could do to change it.

Your body is actually here to gift you the joy of living here on planet earth. Your body is your biggest ally in this life and it wants to contribute to you. You can use and abuse it to your heart's content and it will still get you out of bed in the morning, take a walk when you want, have sex when you desire, and eat the foods you feed it. It is my point of view that your body has more awareness about what would be kind and nurturing to you than you do.

The challenge I see in this reality is that it is a learned habit to control the body without actually asking the body what the body knows.

What if you could ask your body what it knows? What if your body could talk back?

What then?

What isn't working in your body or in your life, is generally an invitation to step into a greater possibility that you don't yet know is available...especially when it comes to the body, it's like the body is inviting you to step into more of your greatness than you previously knew was possible. It wants to invite all the molecules of the universe into the transformation that is actually possible so that a greater force, both inside of you and outside of you can contribute to instigating the magic that is actually possible.

I tell my story so you can use the words that light you up, that give you more information, as a way to listen to the roars and whispers your own body is offering you every day.

True healing is the ability to know that you don't need fixing. You are more brilliant and beautiful and amazing and magnetic then you have been willing to acknowledge. When you begin to acknowledge your magic and gifts, then a different possibility exists.

You can follow your awareness, ask questions, and enjoy the adventure that is you and your body in this lifetime. This reality is programmed to get you to think you need to change who you are, but all those cute quirks and strange thoughts actually create you as the unique being you are.

I've always had the point of view that the abuse and pain and trauma are not wrong. Each experience in this lifetime helped form who I am today. I don't regret any of those cataclysmic events. Each one of those events shaped me into the person I am today. It isn't about changing who we are, so much as it is acknowledging the brilliance.

Healing the things you think you cannot change is about being in allowance of who you are. When you are willing to be you, then what seems like a brick wall becomes an opportunity to acknowledge your brilliance.

You don't need changing, just the way you look at who you are needs to change.

What brilliance is whispering you to play with?

If you didn't need to change who you are, who would you be? What difference could you make on the planet?

This is your invitation to be bold, be you, be the greatness and joy and intensity and magic of you no matter what happens to you and your body.

Would you be willing to acknowledge the greatness of you?

After all, isn't that why you are here?

I wonder what you'll create?

Let the magic begin.

About the Author
KATHERINE McINTOSH

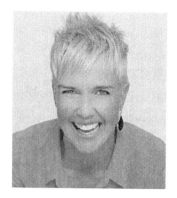

Katherine McIntosh is a Business Coach & Body Intuitive who's traveled the world and worked with performance artists, coaches, musicians, actors, and businesses making a difference on the planet. With a tenacious entrepreneurial spirit, Katherine has built multiple businesses from the ground up to amazing success in a short amount of time using a different kind of approach to business. She is an Access Consciousness® Certified Facilitator, a Motivational Speaker, Business Coach, Mom, and Best Selling Author who desires to show everyone their best and most brilliant selves!

From the age of six, Katherine was fascinated with the human body and it's accompanying psyche. She studied to get her Master's in Somatic Psychology, and also studied physiology, and the systems of the body as well as numerous healing modalities over the last two decades. Katherine studied Shamanism and taught Dance Movement for over 15 years. Her knowledge of the body is quite remarkable. She has a knack for the subtle details of the body and its capacity to heal itself. She believes that almost anything can be uncovered and changed in the body and therefore have an impact on your entire life.

She became aware of healing at a very young age, but shoved her abilities out of her reach due to her Catholic Upbringing. Once Katherine reached her 20s, she could no longer deny there was something she knew about bodies that other people didn't. So she began a quest that would change the course of her life.

She has been working with and on bodies for almost two decades and has a wisdom and light heartedness as well as a piercing ability to hold space and cut to the heart of the matter for some of the most challenging circumstances. Katherine always knew she had a gift with bodies, and at the same time struggled with her own body image until she realized it was her awareness of other bodies that was causing the disruption in her own system. Out of a need to change the way she saw herself, Katherine created the No-Judgment Diet, a 30 day on-line program designed to get you out of judgment in every area of your life, so that you can start to use your talents and abilities to your advantage. Katherine is on a mission to change the way people see themselves, their bodies, healing, food, relationships, money, and their lives in general.

Are you ready for something different? Visit www.katherinemcintosh.com.

Chapter 7

Being for Yourself What You Wish You Got from Others: 4 Keys to Healing

By Heather P. Smith

"Healing is what naturally arises from increasing your awareness." – Gary M. Douglas, founder of Access Consciousness®

Being the kindness, caring, nurturing and gratitude for yourself that you wish you got from other people is a very different way to function. I personally have known it to be the foundation from which healing begins.

What if the choice to be this for yourself is readily available in each moment of every day?

What if you did not need a reason to choose to be kind, caring and nurturing with you?

What if gratitude for you exactly as you are right now opens up the ability to change anything?

What if you could choose it just because you can?

Would you be willing to begin practicing choosing this, even if you don't know how, even if you don't know what kindness, caring, nurturing and gratitude for you really is?

Here is a different approach to healing, and practical steps you can take to begin.

Key 1: Willingness

The desperation and difficulty of not knowing how to handle or change what you have been through, and how to move forward can be daunting. What if you don't have to know how? What if the place to start is to be willing to move forward and change, no matter what it takes?

Just willingness.

Willingness is a magical potency that you already have available if you choose it, if you allow it.

Willingness is; no matter what it takes to change this I will go on the adventure of finding out.

It is an openness that you are willing to let go of your life as it currently is and allow for something else to show up, anything else. It is willing to be different than you have been, to let go of everything you have used to define you. It is being there for yourself and with yourself, in the face of everything. It is having your own back, knowing you will be there for you in all the ways you wish other people were there for you and are not.

With willingness, you have no conditions for the healing and change you are asking for. It can show up however it shows up, in any form. It can show up whenever it shows up, not based on how long it takes, but in the trust that it will, whenever it does.

There is a kind of inner peacefulness and patience for the process that arises when you have the willingness to be, do, have, choose, change and create whatever it takes to have the healing you are seeking.

Your willingness to be in the question of "I wonder what it will take to change this?" and allowing the universe to deliver a possibility for what you are asking to show up is a magical choice you have available right now.

Your willingness to let go of what is, to allow for something different, is key.

Are you willing to have your body feel different in the next five minutes than it does right now?

Are you willing to not have an answer or solution, but instead allow for infinite possibilities?

Are you willing to no longer define yourself based on what has been?

Are you willing to start having a different conversation with yourself, your body and other people?

Your willingness to allow you to be different, to allow your body to be different, to allow your life to be different is a choice you have available right now.

It simply takes you choosing it to have it.

Key 2: Vulnerability

When you are willing to be vulnerable with you, you become vulnerable enough to acknowledge you don't wish to keep living as you have been. When you are vulnerable enough with yourself to be willing to be, do and have whatever it takes to change...the universe goes into action on your behalf to begin delivering what you ask for. The universe shows you how. The universe shows you the steps to take to have what you are asking for. All you must do is step toward what you seek to change. Your willingness to be, do and have whatever it takes to change is that step. That willingness moves you forward. Vulnerability with YOU allows what you are seeking to show up.

Vulnerability with yourself is one of the most powerfully healing capacities and choices you have available to you.

Vulnerability with yourself will give you clarity. Vulnerability with yourself will give you the strength to keep going until you achieve the change and healing you are seeking. Vulnerability with yourself is a way to begin showing up with and for yourself like you wish other people would and do not.

You are the only one who truly knows everything about you, everything you have been through, and everything going on in your inner world. What if you were willing to be present with all of it without a point of view, without any judgment of ANY OF IT being wrong, being right, being bad, being good?

If you choose to be vulnerable with you, all of the judgment drops away. You can look at what is. When you are able to be present with what is, the doors to infinite possibilities for change open. Change is what creates healing. Awareness creates healing.

When you are vulnerable with all the energies of your body and your life; you lose the significance and meaning you or others have given your sickness, disease, disability or limitation and the stuckness of it all unlocks.

So much of the healing you seek becomes possible when you will stand in the face of it all with no barriers and simply receive.

All those energies (and people, and events and awareness) you have been defending against, trying to protect yourself from, stop or avoid become powerless in the face of your vulnerability.

Everything you have been defending against knowing, being, receiving or perceiving become a contribution to the healing you are asking for when you lower your barriers and choose to be totally vulnerable as you and with it.

Key 3: Asking

Have you actually asked for the healing you desire?

Or, have you wished for it, believed you can't have it, believed it is not possible because you can't work out how? Have you been told what you have going on is not curable? What if that is a lie? What if it is just that the doctor, the specialist, the expert or person giving you that point of view does not know how? Don't buy their answer about what is not possible.

Instead ask **"What else is possible that would allow this to change?"**

What would it take to add one hour a day that is just for nurturing, kindness, caring and gratitude for you? How many different things can you choose that embody these qualities?

Not what you have been told is healthy to choose, not what other people say is nurturing, kindness, caring and gratitude...would you be willing to ask yourself what is truly nurturing for you?

Would you be willing to ask yourself what is truly kindness for you?

Would you be willing to ask yourself what is truly caring for you?

Would you be willing to ask yourself what gratitude truly is for you?

What if your point of view about this is different than other people's point of view?

Would you be willing to know what is true for you?

Would you consider choosing what is true for you, even if you do not know any other people who would choose what you choose?

A true question is from the curiosity of wondering what else is possible that you never considered and then to go out in the world, or exploring your inner world from wondering "What is this really?"

A true question is an openness. When you are functioning as the question (and asking questions), you aren't looking for an answer, you are asking for awareness.

By the act of asking a question, an energetic awareness will instantly be available. A cognitive awareness might become available from asking, or it might not. Your awareness of the energies of something is far more useful than a cognitive answer. Be willing to let go of the necessity for a cognitive answer, and instead follow the energy. The energy never lies.

As the question, you are open to noticing things you did not notice before.

You are open to having a different point of view, or even no point of view about what is going on for you. Instead you are in the curiosity of what did I choose that contributed to creating this?

You have a willingness to let go of what you thought was true, and find out what you have not been aware of.

You have a willingness to let go of the definitions of you, the limitations of you and find out what you are capable of that you never allowed before.

One of the best questions for creating and opening up to the healing that is possible is to ask:

What will it take to change this?

Or, **Body, what can I be different that will allow all of this to change?**

Key 4: Gratitude

Gratitude and judgment cannot co-exist.

With the choice to have gratitude for you and everything your life has been up to this point, you can move forward creating a more gentle, nurturing, kind and caring future for yourself.

The choices you make every day are creating your life. Change your choices and you change how your life is showing up. It is a choice to judge. We are taught the correctness of judging, and that judgment will create. Judgment never creates, it only destroys. Every moment you choose gratitude instead of judgment, you invite kindness, caring and nurturing into your life.

What if you are not a judgable offense?

What if you have never chosen wrong?

What if you are not bad?

What if you are not good or right either?

What if just for today, you dropped all your judgments of you and your body? What if just for today you leave your judgments at the door? Don't worry, you can go pick them back up later if you would like to. But, what if just for today you let all those judgments go and instead choose to have gratitude?

What if it is that simple?

Would you allow it to be that easy to have kindness, caring and nurturing for you?

Simply, right now in this moment, drop all the judgment and be grateful for you and your body.

As you are.

Right now.

What if every choice you make today and tomorrow and the day after that and going forward from there could be an ever increasing space of kindness, caring, nurturing and gratitude for you and your body? Would you be willing to allow that for you? Would you be willing to choose that for you?

The choice is yours, my friend.

What will you choose?

About the Author

HEATHER P. SMITH

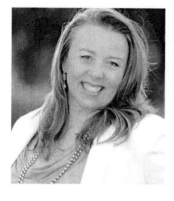

At the age of 21, Heather went on the adventure of healing herself of asthma.

She was told after the first time of having an asthma attack, at age 13, that it was not possible to heal herself, at best she could hope for was managing the symptoms with an inhaler, restricted diet and avoiding those things that might trigger and asthma attack. Maybe she would grow out of it, the doctors told her.

After seven years of living with this she made a demand of herself – no matter what it took she was going to change this! And so it began, the universe went into motion to deliver what she was requesting and demanding of herself to change.

From this, Heather learned about energy. She learned that everything including our thoughts, feelings, emotions, points of view, judgments, choices and actions all have an energy to it. Change the energy and you change how your entire life shows up. She didn't believe it, but she nonetheless explored the possibilities of this and found it to be absolutely true! You really can change the energy and in doing so, it changes everything; including what is not suppose to be changeable.

After a year of daily practice in changing her points of view, letting go of judgment, asking questions and changing the energy of every area of her life and body; she no longer had asthma or any symptoms of asthma of any kind. All the food allergies were gone. All of the asthma attacks were gone. She could run, she could do exercise of any kind and eat anything without it being life threatening.

Heather says; *"I have always been an adventurer and seeker with the insatiable curiosity of wondering 'what else is possible I never considered?'*

The magic of living on this beautiful planet, with a body to play with, the joy of infinite choice to be had and this reality to create - I wonder what could take all of us beyond what we considered possible for healing, uplifting and changing what does not work?

'I can't' has never been real to me. 'What will it take?' is what I live by.

By developing our capacities for being aware of energy and utilizing our natural ability to change the energies we are functioning as, there is no limit to what can be healed and created as our body and our life.

It is our choices we make moment by moment, day by day that create and contribute to everything that is showing up as our life right now. Change your choices and you change how your entire life shows up. This is the potency you have available to you already. Have you been using your capacity for choice for you or against you?"

An Access Consciousness® Facilitator for over nine years now, Heather has found Access to be the easiest modality for changing any area of life. The straight forward simplicity of Access should not be underestimated in its potency and power for transforming energy and providing clarity to those who play with it.

Heather has always been a pragmatist. If she can't use a modality easily in her everyday life and get true and lasting change from its use; she is not interested. Nothing has been more easy to use and simple to apply than the tools of awareness from Access Consciousness®. Empowering people to know that they know is the tag line of Access, and it complements what Heather strives for in facilitation; for a client to know they are the creator of their own life and they have the ability to change anything if they are willing to go on the adventure of discovering what it will take.

Heather is a #1 bestselling author, facilitator, online radio show host, speaker, laughter loving, playful pragmatist...she changes people's lives.

www.heathersmith.accessconsciousness.com
www.endingptsd.com
www.heatherpsmith.com
www.thegoodgirlsguidetobeingwrong.com

Chapter 8

The Kind Whispers
of Healing

By Sylvia Puentes

There is something new in my world. There is a whisper of something different. There is a whisper of something that perhaps I've never put into words until now – THE ENERGY OF HEALING and what I know about what that is for me.

I was not one who considered herself a healer before. You see, I have no medical background, no medical certificate or even alternative medicine experience. And yet, there is a whisper, a gentle tap on the shoulder, saying ..."Hey, you are a healer, it just doesn't look like you think it does."

I suppose I have defined a healer to be someone who is educated in medicine; someone who knows anatomy, physiology, gynecology, kinesiology...all of those "Ologies", someone who can pronounce those long words and someone who can create change in the body with the use of medicine and or knowledge of other healing tools. These are all very interesting points of view I am discovering I have had and never acknowledged. Funny, is it possible that our point of view limits what we are willing to receive and acknowledge? What if what we actually know does not fit that belief, thought or paradigm? I wonder...

So, this chapter begins with a question: What have you defined healing that it is not, that if you didn't define it as such, would allow you to open up to your healing capacities beyond this reality?

What have you defined healing to be for you? Some say that healing is the act of being cured. And often it's being cured by someone or something outside of you. What if healing is a choice and something you can be that cannot only change your issue, but that can change your systems and someone else's world as well.

This is not about giving you answers or telling you how to heal. It is rather an exploration for you to tap into what it is that you know, and perhaps, just maybe, allow you to tap into and begin to acknowledge the gift of healing you may have and are. Would you be willing to explore that?

Growing up with a Curandera

A *Curandera* is a traditional Native healer or shaman found in the United States and Mexico.

As I look back at my younger years, it's interesting that I never acknowledged the alternative healing methods I grew up with. As a first generation Mexican American, I grew up in Northern California with my grandparents and many uncles and aunts nearby. I have many memories of my grandmother, Mama Chilo, whether it was an ear ache or a stomach ache, she would go into her back yard and pick an herb and quickly make a remedy. She had planted herbs all around her garden that she knew were available to ease pain, bruises, rashes, sore muscles, ear aches, stomach aches.

It wasn't until years later I acknowledged the wealth of knowledge she had with plants. As a young teenager there was almost resistance to her "crazy herbs" or that they were used because there was a lack of money. So as I resisted seeing the value. I longed to be like everyone else and have a teaspoon of some over-the-counter medicine. What craziness!

I was probably six or seven years old when my mother took me to visit another family *Curandera* for a much more serious ailment. I apparently had a stomach issue. For some reason I was eating, but not gaining weight, and apparently I was too thin to be healthy. Clearly in their eyes something was wrong with me because I was not plumping up like all the other kids. I recall the late night as I walk in to this unknown house. We were greeted by ladies I had seen before, but did not know very well. They walked me into a room where I was asked to lay down so they could massage my stomach. Apparently I had something stuck or something that needed to be removed so I could gain weight. After the rubbing of my stomach, I was taken in the kitchen where the other woman had cooked up a concoction that did not smell very good. I was given this cup to drink and told I needed to drink it all. Yuck! I recall smelling and tasting cooked onion, orange peels, garlic and who knows what else. So guess what happened next! I quickly plumped up to make sure I didn't return to that remedy again. Apparently, I had been healed.

What if healing is a choice?

What if healing was the ability to change something. Some people call changing the unchangeable or impossible as miracles? Do miracles truly exist?

What do you know?

I was first introduced to Energy Healing by one of my aunts. She introduced me to the idea that I could perceive energy. She showed me that my body had information to share and that it could guide me through a simple muscle testing give me a yes or no to questions. I was definitely intrigued, I was intrigued that I could communicate with my body, I was intrigued that I could begin to not only perceive energy, when the energy shifted or changed and that I had actually been aware of energy all my life and just never had words for it.

A few years after that I discovered Access Consciousness®, energy work that I could use to change all areas of life. For the first time, I started to acknowledge that with a gentle touch healing could occur. I learned that by tapping in to energy, space and consciousness, I could change anything. We could do it on our own or have someone invite us to the change. Yet, it was up to us to be willing to receive the invitation and choose the change.

A few years ago, a mother brought her nine-year-old son to see me. He had been having some trouble at school, dietary issues, and some classmate issues. I remember opening the door and seeing his kind face. There in front of me stood a sweet being, with a soft smile on his face and so much ease and trust. At a glance, I could 'diagnose' no problem, other than what I just described, which made him very different. Without many questions he lay down to receive a session of Access Bars®. This is a hands-on energy work that consists of 32 points on your head which, when gently touched, effortlessly and easily release thoughts, feelings, emotions and beliefs that are creating what isn't working in your life. The mother had also received this non-invasive process only a few hours before him. She now quietly sat about six feet away from her son.

The young boy soon began to have sensations in his body. As I walked him through a short exercise, the sensations moved to another part of his body and then moved again and began to lighten up and almost disappear. I recall him sit up after his session with big wide open eyes, look at his mother and say, "And people said there was no such thing as magic, I always knew there was magic". He had so much joy in acknowledging what he called magic, the ability to move and change something.

So what does magic and healing mean to you?

The gift of touch

There are studies that show infants who suffer from touch deprivation do not thrive and grow at normal healthy rates. Is it possible that touch can be a generative energy that contributes to healthy growth? I recall few memories of being cuddled or held by my parents. And yet when they did give a little scratch on the head or play with my hand, it meant so much. There was some kind of connection being created with each touch.

I have discovered that there are many interesting perspectives in the world about what healing is. Growing up in a Catholic family, I often heard stories about a man who walked on water, brought people up from the dead and healed any disease simply with a touch or even his presence. However, there was still this sense that this healing capacity was only possible for the chosen ones.

In the last five years, I have discovered an entire new reality for healing. I have been practicing the tools and body processes of Access Consciousness®. I have discovered or re-discovered so much about myself and my own capacities through this work that I now share with people around the world. You see, I was never empowered to know that I know something about anything, really. I was never asked the question, "What do you know?"

Have you ever been asked?

Have you ever received the gift of a touch?

Have you ever been hugged by someone, and as you received their hug, you could perceive something changing, you could perceive their kindness and all your resistance fall away? I have, and it has been such a gift to know that this is possible.

What else do I know?

After years of work with people of all ages I discovered few other magical elements to healing that seemed at times to be overlooked. They may be overlooked because they seem too simple or insignificant, or perhaps because they may not be able to be measured scientifically. None the less, I have seen the contribution to change these elements are in people's health and lives. These are: Kindness, Allowance and Joy.

What I have begun to observe and acknowledge in everything I do, is the gift in people's world when I am present, the space of allowance for them to be and choose whatever it is they choose. It is as if this space allows them to drop their guard and not fight to prove they are right about whatever they have decided about their body, their issue, and begin to perceive a different possibility and open up to the willingness to change it. How this happens I don't know exactly, other than their choice to let it go begins to change it all.

What if your kindness is more potent than you think? What if your kindness can melt away what seems unchangeable? Would you be willing to be it and receive it?

What do you know?

As approach the end of this chapter, I wonder what you have perceived, I wonder what new questions you have, I wonder what healing capacity you have, that you have now been invited to see and receive. Thank you for reading and thank you for who you be on this planet. What if each one of us is a gift that can create a difference by being as different as we truly be?

About the Author
SYLVIA PUENTES

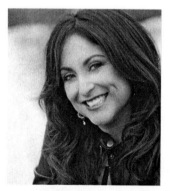

As a bilingual #1 bestselling author, Access Consciousness® Certified Facilitator, Empowerment Coach, International Speaker and Radio Show host, Sylvia Puentes contributes to people of all ages by sharing tools and techniques that can transform any area of life. Her joyful, insightful and kind presence is filled with ease and allowance as she works with individuals and groups to clear limiting blocks and open up the doors to infinite possibilities for a different reality.

She has been using the Access Consciousness® tools to create a life and living filled with ease, joy and infinite possibilities and is now sharing this with the world. Today she is traveling around the world sharing her vision of how empowering people to know that they know creates success in life; school, work and home. Her desire is to reach as many people as possible, in person, print, radio and television and inspire them to live a life with Ease, Joy and Glory.

If you are willing to explore something different, clear limitations and choose to receive more of YOU and the gift you be to the world than tune in and playfully turn everything that's not working for you upside down and ignite the radiant energy of YOU.

For more about Sylvia Puentes go here:

www.sylviapuentes.accessconsciousness.com
www.siendoladona.com

Chapter 9

The Healing Energy of Mediumship and Feng Shui

By Diane Hiller

The field of healing has been a lifelong interest for me. I began as a Licensed Practical Nurse and moved forward to other areas over a 20-year period. This me to my current combination of being a Psychic Medium, Medical Intuitive, Licensed Psychotherapist, and Certified Black Sect Tibetan Buddhist Feng Shui Master.™

I now work predominately with energy on many levels. As a student of Feng Shui, we were taught that any healer was only as good as their own degree of spiritual practice. During my own healing journey, my investigations have led me to use many alternative practices for my own evolvement

125

and I continue to do so. They have included: Reiki, Past Life Regressions, Soul Retrieval, Extraction Healing, and Journey work into each of my own Chakra systems. I'm a big a fan of Shamanism.

Soul or spiritual evolvement and healing to me is a process, not an event. My beliefs encompass integrative medicine and that all dis-ease manifests in the etheric before it becomes physical. However, at that point it needs to be dealt with in traditional ways. Modern medicine has many wonderful options.

My focus here though, is on how I have learned to work with energy in my own practice, describing each aspect of how I do and what I do.

Mediumship

Many of my clients ask me after a session, "How do you do this? This a must just be gift right? How can you possibly know the things you know?" Some of this I can answer and some I learn as my consciousness expands. Aware of my abilities as a very young child, I'm not clear what it feels like not to be psychic.

The gifts in my family are intergenerational on the female side.

As many of you know, all mediums are also psychic but not all psychics are mediums; I am both. Being a medium means you are able to connect with a specific energy called a disincarnate. While reading as a medium, one is merely a conduit for energy to come through me to speak with someone who has died. Never really knowing who is going to show up, I will often connect with the person the client is hoping to hear from, yet someone else entirely may show up. This is the soul in pure energy form, at its own specific vibration. It is like tuning into a specific radio station. I know they are there because I will see what I call a light body. In person, they often walk right through the door with my client.

I read, for the most part, with my eyes closed. During this process I will be shown a certain image of the body along with receiving information through my other abilities of: clairvoyance, (to see), clairaudience, (to hear) claircognizance, (to know) and clairsentience, (to feel.) For example, male and female energy just *feels* different. Or I will simply be told this is a male or female. I may see a head or figure shaped exactly as the person was when they were alive. Other areas may be highlighted and I will hear and hear words like, brain tumor, stroke, and so on. Empathically my own body may feel a sharp or sudden sense of what went wrong, or my hands may move of their own accord to touch an area of my body. Specific other information, which I call qualifiers, may also come through such as: month of birth or death, specific dates or ages, recent events, or current happenings that are specifically meaningful to the client. This is called Evidential Mediumship.

I am sure all mediums have similar as well as different ways they interpret symbols. It is my understanding that these symbols are given to us by our own guides or our personal oracle. They can't be replicated or copied.

At the beginning of any kind of reading, I start in sacred space with a psychic energetic connection by asking that the client take three deep breaths and blow them in to the phone or the room. After this I am then flooded with colors which have reliably come to mean certain things to me: red means health issues, working in health care, or relationship issues. Light blue is job issues, another shade of blue as a line visualized between two people is a strong karmic tie. Black indicates depression, money problems, selfishness, anxiety or some form of negativity. Green is something very new, if combined with red it is often a new relationship or birth. Slanted energy in a certain direction is someone who is lying to my client. While seeing all of these colors, or just few at a time, I get the reason why my client has come to see me before they say a word. The colors shift and change and are fluid in the reading, which also has its own set of interpretations. Then the reading proceeds go on from there, with my guides or departed loved ones giving me information. Many times I also see direct images of a property that the client lives on or is moving to. Additionally, I have seen detailed crime scenes, certain objects, pieces of jewelry, and things that are very specific to the client. Each reading is different. On occasion I begin to speak very quickly and am in a light trance state, when this happens I am hearing the information at the same time as the client.

Mediumship is healing in the sense that the client knows

for sure with whom I am speaking. These sessions tend to be quite emotional, often bringing a sense of closure, acceptance, resolution, and peace for all parties. Things may have been left unsaid; the client wants to know that their loved one is "okay." In fact, "Are they okay?" is the most frequent question I am asked, especially if the death was recent. Receiving messages of love, validation, or knowing what is going on in the person's life are very powerful. Not all readings are serious; some relatives come though that turn the session in to something that left the client laughing in recognition of the person's intact personality and things they were saying. A reading can be life altering. I myself have had several which have had this impact on my own life.

Medical Intuitive Work

My background as a nurse has helped me put energetic feelings in to symptomatology and well as medical terms. During this type of reading information comes though clairvoyance, or clairaudience, but of late I have been guided to use my right hand to scan a person's body. This can be done in person or over the phone. While moving my hand I am guided to stop at certain places to discuss what is going on, and can often feel where there has been surgery or ongoing issues. The center of my palm will become energetically very hot where there is a significant issue that needs to be looked into. I tell my clients what information comes from my guides, and I always refer them back to their MD to have things investigated.

Feng Shui

Feng Shui is all about energy. When engaged in a consult I am looking at the nine energy centers of the home and what is or is not present. How is the "chi" or life force moving though the home? There is an analysis of water flow, electrical issues, door, bed and, fireplace placements as well as structural issues. A Feng Shui consult of your home is a microscopic view in a macrocosmic field of live energy. Whatever issues may be present in your life at the moment will show up in your floor plan.

There are nine energy centers that are present in the home as a whole, in each room and on the outside property. The areas are related to: career, knowledge and spirituality, family and the past, wealth, reputation, relationships, children and creativity the future, and benefactors. Assessing if the energy is blocked, absent, moving too fast or slow, or simply not present due to structural issues then leads to suggested adjustments. Energetic adjustments and the use of intention through spiritual empowerments to these areas can rapidly bring about desired changes and results.

Space Clearing and Blessing/Spirit Removal

As a further area of training in the program, we learned to deal with unwanted energy in a home or place of business. More and more of late I find myself being called to homes to remove intrusive energies. There may be a spirit that is stuck and has not crossed over, other unwanted energy may have to do with predecessor chi or what occurred in the home with prior owners. The most common causes are domestic violence, substance abuse, or a murder or suicide connected to the property. When I receive a call for this type of work and have accepted a deposit, it is common for me to have disrupted sleep the night before. It is though they know I am coming. After parking outside of the home, I stand outside for several minutes and almost always "see" where the energetic problem lies. My eyes and body will be drawn to the problem areas. I then will go into the home talk to the owner (s) for a few moments and then do a walk though of the home. I will immediately feel in my solar plexus where the energy is most prominent.

A typical energy clearing will proceed in the following way. I combine several different traditions when doing a space clearing. I start by using a sacred shamanic drum made with the shaman I work with; it has been spiritually empowered. It is only used for space clearing and journeywork and not for drumming circles. I do seven rounds each in the four directions throughout the home. This will break up any psychometric energy that is held in the walls. I then go back to the areas where I felt the most disruption and chant scared mantras for as long as it takes to clear the energy. When chant I am asking light beings to come in to assist with the removal of these energies. I often will use Buddhist mantra in rounds of 108. Nine is the number of completion in Feng Shui. I may use six or more different mantra depending on what I am guided to use. The seed syllables of these mantras are very powerful. I then mix and burn a combination of sage, tobacco and sweet grass, as used in an Indian burial ritual. This mixture is very effective is removing negativity. The windows are open or all faucets in the home are running to take out the energy.

Then I will adjust the external chi with a Traditional Rice Blessing. This is a mixture of white rice, cinnabar, and alcohol that is above 100 proof, such as Grave's Wood Alcohol or Bacardi 151, which has also been spiritually empowered by mantra. The reason for the high alcohol content is that the vibrational rate of the alcohol has the ability to overcome incorporeal spirits that may be wandering around. One handful is thrown outward in the four cardinal directions to "feed the hungry ghosts," one handful in thrown downward in the four directions to plant the seeds of luck or auspicious chi, three handfuls are thrown upward with the intention to raise the energetic vibration of the property.

Once the property has been cleared inside and outside, I then empower quartz crystal with spiritual energy to create a grid of light in the home and on the property as protection from further issues.

Working with and studying energy is my life's passion and purpose. I feel very honored to do the work I do each day.

About the Author
DIANE HILLER

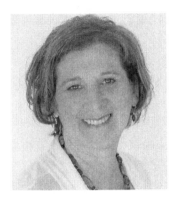

Diane Hiller is a Psychic Medium, Medical Intuitive, Psychotherapist and Certified Feng Shui Master and #1 bestselling author. She is an innovative expert in the field of metaphysics and is widely recognized in her field. She is a former nurse and Phi Beta Kappa, receiving both her undergraduate degree in Psychology and Master's in Clinical Social Work at The University of Connecticut. Diane has extensively studied both Buddhism and Shamanism and received certification as a Black Sect Tibetan Buddhist Feng Shui Master™. This professional training program was originally formed at the request and under the guidance the late His Holiness Professor Thomas Lin Yun, a world-renowned expert in Feng Shui. She is a member of the International Feng Shui Guild. She has been featured in The Top 100 Psychic and Astrologers in America by Paulette Cooper and Paul Noble, in the 2015 Best Psychics Mediums and Lightworkers in the United States, by Maximillian de Lafayette, as well as The National and International Rank of The World's Best Lightworkers 2014-2015 by Maximillien de Lafayette. She was ranked internationally by popular vote as within the top 10 as a Psychic, Psychic Medium, Feng Shui Master and Life Coach. She was inducted, for life, in to the Lightworker's World Hall of Fame on December 11, 2014.

Diane's psychic gifts were evident at the age of nine. They fully awakened during her personal healing journey, through the study of shamanism and chakra journeywork, then following two very powerful kundalini openings. She is founder and owner of Elemental Empowerments, LLC, in Litchfield, Connecticut and combines the arts of Mediumship, Psychotherapy, Feng Shui, and spiritual life coaching in her professional practice. Diane's educational background and skills give her insight and understanding of your life challenges and her spiritual toolbox is full of abilities to work with you on numerous energetic levels. It is an honor and privilege for Diane to be of service to you. Diane reads locally in her Litchfield office and does phone readings both in the USA and Internationally. Her contact information is as follows:

Phone: (860) 601-1263
Email: dianehiller@optonline.net
Website: www.ElementalEmpowerments.com
Facebook: https://www.facebook.com/
DianeHillerPsychicMedium?ref=hl

Chapter 10

Simple Natural Health

By Donna LaBar

My 12-year-old daughter Monica and I clung together sobbing as the oncologist quietly left Monica's hospital room. We thought Monica had a strange virus that she couldn't shake. Two months went by and my once athletic, witty, practical jokester slowly melted into a world of 24-hour care, blood tests, and IVs. Now we knew what it was. It had a name and with that came the horrifying truth of how life can change in an instant.

Monica was diagnosed on November 24, 1998, with Acute Myloid Leukemia, AML. She went from complaining of hip and joint pain in the summer, to flu-like symptoms in early October, to total hospitalization by the end of November. Receiving the diagnosis went something like this: "Monica, you have a cancer of your blood that is very aggressive. It appears you have had it for three to six months. It has shown itself to be a terminal cancer in the elderly population. We can give you chemotherapy, large doses, like a sledge hammer to your system. You may not make it through the first two weeks of this treatment. We believe at this stage you may have two weeks to live without treatment. In addition, you also have a blood-clotting disorder, which makes taking chemotherapy very dangerous. We must try to establish if your ability to clot can be corrected or chemotherapy is not an option. I will be sending in members of our team to talk about all of this with you and your Mom."

Then the doctor quietly exits the room.

Back up to my late teen years. In September 1975, I get a co-operative education job through my school in a school-to-work program. I had been a business major in high school and was happy to get a job as a starter legal secretary for a local law firm. I was there about a year when they hired a new attorney, fresh out of law school, and she and I became fast friends. I lived in northern rural Pennsylvania and she had grown up in West Chester, just outside of Philadelphia.

On weekends, we would make the trek to visit her parents.

They were eclectic couple. She had been a nurse but left the field to raise their children and he was a chemical engineer. I will call them Jo and Al. They enjoyed their gardens, reading and the art of conversation. We quickly became friends. They helped me create a huge lovely rock garden and taught me a lot about botanicals. A few years into the friendship, Al was experiencing illness and was diagnosed with stomach cancer. He was around 60 years old at the time. They quickly determined that he needed to have his stomach removed. Of course, there weren't many alternatives 30 years ago, so he went for the surgery even though the prognosis was not encouraging.

He made it through the surgery and decided to use his knowledge of chemistry and

apply it to healing himself. With the normal digestion process unavailable, taking enzymes and supplements became a way of life in order to get proper nutrition. Jo helped him with her interest in natural foods and cooking. During this time, I became close to Al and was totally intrigued by his studies and discoveries regarding nutritional and natural healing.

He was like a mad scientist, and I was the inquisitive apprentice. He would come up with recipes and formulas for things that would correct illnesses, mostly for his friends and family. I would help him in his quest to find products that were already on the market that were similar to his original recipes so we could direct friends where to find something that would help them. I learned so much and started to maintain my health with holistic approaches. I would research different opinions, data and studies, and would discuss them with Al, always looking for that which made the most sense and that which was the most reasonable approach for the common individual. Al taught me so much and lived a wonderful full life, just passing on recently at the age of 93.

My fascination with natural healing and the discoveries I had with Al about the body's abilities to repair itself were part of my life for 20 years or so by the time Monica was ill. The purpose for my inquisitive studies and passion for alternative healing quickly snapped into focus with her cancer diagnosis. I worked with her oncologists combining conventional treatment with alternative approaches. We left no stone unturned. Monica and I tried many different things to help her mind, body and spirit during this time. We believed she could make it through this, not easily, but still attainably, just one day at a time. She would be our miracle. She healed, and is alive today, quite vibrant and in her 20s.

I hold the strong belief in healing, and in healing miracles.

There have been, not just one, but millions of cases of miraculous healing documented through the centuries! So why can't that be you? If you were suddenly scratched today, in a few days the scratch would be scabbed over and in a few weeks it would for the most part be gone. This is part of the miracle - the body not only can heal itself, healing is truly a part of its design! Supporting the body's complex bio chemical ability to heal is not difficult, in fact it's easy!

Your body does all the complicated stuff automatically when given the right ingredients.

Start today. Your body will gladly cooperate. After all, if you give it exactly what it needs when it needs it, you will never find anything on the planet that operates as keenly and efficiently as the human body. Our body, with over 50 trillion cells, will completely replace every cell in a year. The body has the amazing ability to maintain a temperature of 98.6 degrees, maintain an alkaline/acid pH balance of 7.365, regulate blood sugar levels, regulate fluids, make enzymes and hormones, digest and absorb nutrients to nourish cells, regenerate healthy cells, anticipate what is good and bad for us, plus remove toxins and waste. The body is fully equipped to recover from illness or injury and heal itself. The most amazing pharmacy is the human body!

Our health is influenced by three environments which we provide. The first environment is built by the food we eat to nourish our cells to maintain normal body functions. Second, the thoughts we think that either make us feel great or make us ill. And, third, our surroundings, where we live, work, play and create. Our choices and how, good or bad, they predict much of our health experiences and future.

How we nourish the body is very important in relation to what it has to offer back to us for mental and physical leverage. Like a computer: garbage in, garbage out. We must have some basic knowledge of good maintenance for the body to get the most out of it. It's exciting for me to provide some cool information that has helped many people make all difference in their lives!

One very important fact that few know about is that our body needs to maintain a pH balance between 7.35 and 7.45 to remain healthy. When we are born our body is alkaline and as we are exposed to the elements like food, environment and stresses, the body can become acidic. This simple fact is one of the most common reasons we see so much illness today. Once the body drops below 7, an acidic state, health begins to decline and eventually disease is present. This process can be slow and goes from a state of just uncomfortable bouts of inflammation, heartburn or acid reflux, insomnia, etc., in which case the individual will take over-the-counter drugs such as pain killers, stomach and digestive aids, stool softeners and laxatives or sleep aids. Eventually, it will be necessary to step the process of decline to the level of more complex medicines from a doctor for worsening symptoms. The person doesn't look at their diet or lifestyle or thoughts at this point, they just consider this normal non-life threatening health issues or a stage of aging. As the body continues with no sustenance for maintaining normal alkaline/acid levels, inflammatory issues ensue and diseases like cancer, diabetes, MS, lupus, arthritis, fibromyalgia, etc. become common diagnosis.

Cancer for instance does not grow in an alkaline base, however it does grow easily in an acidic environment. It is my belief that if an individual is trying to prevent or slow an ailment or disease, or is receiving treatment for cancer, it is very important to provide the body with a diet that is 75 percent alkaline foods and 25 percent acid foods to support the body through the process to recovery. This can be as easy as looking at an alkaline/acid food chart and making choices that leave your plate filled with 75 percent of alkaline-forming foods you have chosen and 25 percent of acid- forming foods. There is a basic alkaline/acid food chart available on my website, www.DonnaLaBar.com, to help you make this assessment. Alkaline foods are not necessarily known with basic common sense, so a chart will be helpful until you are comfortable. For instance, a lemon is acidic in its natural state, however, once ingested becomes alkaline-forming and is therefore and excellent choice. On the other hand, a banana is alkaline in its natural state because of its high potassium content, however, becomes acid-forming once ingested because of its' high sugar content.

Alkalinity in the body happens as a result of the mineral content in our foods. The primary minerals that have an alkalizing effect are calcium, iron, magnesium, manganese and potassium. In order to support the body to keep the alkaline state, eating foods rich in the primary minerals is the key. These minerals are all very important for pH balance and all of them have different health benefits. It is imperative to have a diet rich in plant-based, low sugar content foods to provide the balance needed for the proper function of all of our organs and natural healing. Our complex bio chemical system creates our enzymes and hormones, fluctuates our fluids, runs our organs and repairs and replaces cells non-stop, gets what it needs to perform from our food and water.

If you are curious to know where you stand, buy a pack of alkaline test strips for urine testing. Tear off a strip and dip it in your urine stream and check the color it turns again the chart provided with the strips. Generally a yellow strip reveals acidic urine and a medium/dark green color strip is alkaline. It is best to check urine as opposed to saliva because it's best to test after the body has ingested the food.

I mentioned environments that influence our alkaline/acid balance. Your food choices do have a huge impact on health and so do your thoughts. Anxious thoughts and worry naturally make the body produce cortisol and adrenaline. These secretions are acidic. If this state becomes constant, or a way of life, the individual can experience acidity and possibly hormonal problems in spite of a good diet. Another place that acidity can show up in spite of a good diet is through extreme exercise. I have read about soda doping, where an athlete will drink water with baking soda (sodium bicarbonate) to get their lactic acid level down after an extreme demand on their body from physical exercise. It is said that it can have a significant effect on endurance and speed due to the alkalizing effect of the blood pH. The goal of all of this is to create and support the perfect environment in our body to function properly. This supports our body's ability to utilize and produce enzymes.

Without Enzymes We Would Not Be Alive

Enzymes, without them, we would not be alive. We need them to eat and breathe.

Our body does produce a staggering number of different types of enzymes, which is awesome, except it does not do this indefinitely and especially without the right conditions. A poor diet and accelerated aging can cause the decline in the body's ability to produce enzymes. The more conscious a person is about getting enzymes in their diet, the more healthy and energetic they become. Enzyme richness will dramatically slow the aging process and the progression of disease.

When food is cooked beyond 116 degrees Fahrenheit, the enzymes are destroyed in the process. Eating uncooked, unprocessed food is the best way to ensure your body is getting a steady supply of enzymes. Having enzymes active in food allows it to digest easily without as much work for the body because the food contains the necessary enzymes for digestion. A change as simple as being mindful to eat a live component with every meal will quickly improve digestion, reduce acid and provide better elimination. As a result of improving the digestive process, you are rewarded with more energy and increased mental clarity. The great news is that you experience all of this fairly quickly. The body responds graciously when it has the right materials to work with.

There is a caveat to this, not all foods can be utilized for their full nutritional potential without being cooked. For instance, carbohydrates (starches) are a good example. In the cooking process, the starch molecule is broken down with heat and water, called gelatinization, making it more enjoyable and easier for the body to get nutrients from it. Foods like grains, root vegetables, corn, dried beans and peas become edible and provide absorbable nutrients by being cooked. The body creates the enzymes necessary for the digestion of these carbohydrates.   It may be necessary to supplement with digestive enzymes if your body has trouble digesting foods that are important in your diet. Since enzymes not only help with digestion and absorption, they also assist in elimination, it is imperative we get enzymes in some fashion to support our health.

The Importance of Elimination (Good Poop)

I mentioned elimination and I can't responsibly discuss proper digestion without covering the importance of removing waste and toxins from the body as steadily and as regularly as we put food in for nourishment. The best rule of thumb I believe is that you should have a bowel movement after each meal, so you may go three times a day or more. It's important not to have prolonged diarrhea or constipation as neither is normal and both can lead to serious illness. With diarrhea, crucial nutrients may not be absorbed during digestion leaving the body malnourished in spite of the fact that you are eating regularly. Constipation can be equally debilitating. The waste after digestion and inhalation is full of bacteria, toxins and pollutants that need to exit regularly.

Constipation is a condition created when the body, dehydrated, pulls all of the fluid out of the waste or stool to use in our blood and lymph system to maintain the amount of fluid necessary to function. It's a survival skill on the part of the resourceful body responding to the immediate crisis. Of course this fluid is septic and a poor source of fluid in the long term. Without proper hydration, this can go on for a long time and slowly deteriorating your health.

Proper hydration and fiber in the diet is so important for the elimination process. Keeping the body hydrated so it can pump blood to the organs and toxins can clear through our lymphatic system is vital. Fiber helps the waste to move on through the body and is eliminated with ease. A constant supply of water intake and good roughage at meal times will keep these matters in check or keep you "regular" as the saying goes. It may be necessary to create new routines that include keeping fresh water close by at all times. I have found that I easily drink water all day with a supply with me in my car and at my desk. Not hydrating leaves you feeling very tired by the afternoon. When I'm feeling sluggish it's my natural alarm that my body is low on fluids, I reach for a big glass of water and amazingly get energized.

Balancing Your Blood Sugar

Another diet related issue with energy is the roller coaster ride your blood sugar takes if your diet is not balanced. A balanced diet consists of carbohydrates, proteins and fats. Proteins and fats allow the body to create tissue and insulation, so you must eat some lean protein and healthy fats. Carbohydrates provide calories used to make energy. The energy produced from carbohydrates is used for our normal everyday body functions like movement, heartbeat, breathing and digesting. There are two categories of carbohydrates, simple and complex.

Simple carbohydrates get there name because they are simple sugars that do not have a lot of nutritional value, digest quickly and therefore enter the bloodstream fast. Some examples of simple carbs are table sugar, white flour and any products with these ingredients as well as honey, molasses, jelly, jam, fruit juices, fruit, flavored yogurts, chocolate, soda and packaged cereals, just to name a few of the most popular. The fast pace of current times have left most of the population chasing their energy slumps throughout the day with caffeine and simple carbohydrates. This is the ride that takes you to the bad lands!

Caffeine gives the adrenaline rush and simple sugars quickly raise your blood sugar for a short time leaving you feeling awake and charged for an instant; then the big descend to low blood sugar, which leaves you extremely tired and wanting a big nap. You can easily get off this ride. Eliminate simple carbohydrates, they are energy thieves! Your addiction to caffeine will gradually disappear as the experience of intense fatigue from swaying blood sugar is eliminated. In addition to the feeling of exhaustion, huge peeks and valley with blood sugar is just the start of sliding down a slippery slope with your health. Obesity, pre diabetes and diabetes are out of control in many societies, a huge problem for the United States. Avoiding simple carbs and becoming mindful of how you feel when you eat, will bring you closer to enjoying solid, stable good health. Food should make you feel neither charged nor exhausted. Start paying attention, being mindful of how you feel a half hour after a meal or snack.

Complex carbohydrates on the other hand are important in our diet and act as fuel and give us energy. They have a more complex chemical makeup, a complex of sugars made up of fiber, minerals and vitamins. Complex carbs take longer to digest so they enter the blood slower, and do not cause the ups and downs in energy of simple carbohydrates. Complex carbs are found in vegetables and whole grains, examples of them are beans, broccoli, celery, legumes, lentils, spinach, yams and zucchini. Complex carbs give you the most bang for your buck so to speak. You can eat them in abundance without adding a lot of calories, and they provide loads of vitamins and nutrients along with more hydration and fiber to aid in digestion and elimination. Our spark or energy is fueled by enzymes, minerals and water. Your diet should be loaded with alkaline complex carbohydrates. This will keep your light shining brightly.

Experiencing Happiness

Enjoying happiness and feeling optimistic should be a normal part of life. We are meant to live in harmony and cooperation, not competing and fighting. Part of our internal health is what we eat but the other half is what we think. As I mentioned earlier, we have three environments that influence our health. Eating properly is half the battle, but thinking healthy is another huge element to wellness. Bad thoughts, worrying and monkey mind bring on stress, anxiety, sadness and sometimes depression. All of this is extremely hard on your body. When you are stressed the body automatically creates hormones to deal with this threatening information the body senses. That is our fight or flight response, still keenly in place as part of our complex bodily functions to protect us from danger.

Now you don't need this to flee from dinosaurs as our ancestors did, but it does signal you every single time that something feels wrong, sounds wrong or smells wrong to you. If you could just become aware of what makes you happy and what makes you sad or frightened, then simply embrace more of the first and avoid the later, you would be doing a momentous boost to every cell in your body and would make a significant improvement in your overall health and life. Some professionals do muscle testing, applied kinesiology, to see if your body tests weak or strong to a product, idea or question. This is an amazing way to experience how your body instinctively knows what it believes is good for it and what is bad.

Getting in touch with this and beginning to honor yourself by acknowledging what does not make you happy and correcting this is just as important as you being mindful to eat healthier to feel the energy that is provided by your food, thus make this connection of how what is in your mind and body can fuel you or make you wilt. It may be as simple as starting to say no to things or people that no longer support or serve who you are and what makes you hum along nicely.

Addressing these issues can be equally or more difficult than getting rid of the morning java with a bagel, but the rewards are staggering and a must if you are going to enjoy total wellness. Once you have committed to solve the hardest issues, so many things will fall into place automatically. You will feel better, so you will eat better and exercise willingly, relax more and sleep peacefully. This is the cycle to strive for.

Good Sleep

Sleeping really well and waking up refreshed is an imperative part of healthy living. When you sleep, a nice full, long, uninterrupted sleep, your body heals and repairs itself. This is the important part of the equation that helps keep you from illness and disease as well as giving you prolonged youthfulness and a creative active mind. When the mind and the diet are a mess, good sleep can become impossible. You must work through this and there are many things to try. You may need to try them all, but don't stop until you have conquered any sleep troubles you have.

First, make sure you are tired! Just being exhausted mentally isn't enough to get you a good night of sleep, you need to be physically tired as well. Even if you are not mentally exhausted, you should get physical exercise to promote good sleeping. Get in the habit of at least a walk in the morning, at lunchtime or after dinner. The more aggressive the stroll you take the better. Breathe in fully to force good oxygen into your cells and stretch a bit too if you think of it. All of this gets you a valuable good sleep with a fresher feeling when you wake. Don't avoid a chance to do physical work, our lives have become way to sedentary. Take the stairs, run to the post office, in fact run your errands! We say we are out to run our errands, but we always take the car! Push yourself whenever you can. Use it or lose it – they were not kidding. Remember, you are doing all of this for delicious healthy sleep and total overall wellness.

The most typical things to help sleep are to take a warm bath in Epsom salts and a bit of baking soda and relax with soft light and music. Clear your mind and prepare for a good night of rest. It may also help to have an herb tea that is offered as a sleep aid such as chamomile tea, or warm milk with a hint of nutmeg (my grandmother's favorite). Minerals such as calcium and magnesium also help with sleep. Taking your calcium with magnesium supplement at bedtime is good for sleeping and also providing your body with minerals to assist in the repair of your body during slumber.

Other supplements like melatonin or 5-htp can also be helpful. The choice of vitamin or vitamins can depend on your reason for insomnia. Melatonin is the most well known for helping people get rest. It is a hormone that your body may slow or quit making cause trouble with your internal clock. The dosage really can vary a lot depending on the individual. It's best to start with a small dosage and work your way up if you are trying this supplement. If you are not taking enough, you may experience vivid dreams or even nightmares, so you will know if you need more. If you wake up short of a full night of sleep take another and it will ease you back to sleep easily. The 5-htp is the precursor to L-tryptophan which raises the serotonin level. It makes you feel better overall and helps calm your mind. I know individuals that take 50 to 100 mg in the morning and 50 to 100 mg at night and this seems to steady them through their day and give them a peaceful night of sleep.

One of my favorites is reading to get ready to sleep. I also like listening to an audio book, and sometimes I use headset to tune into vibrational beats and tones to help me get into a deep sleep. If you are a poor sleeper, don't give up. Keep making the necessary changes in your life to get the rest you need. It may take a few changes or many, take just one step at a time.

Making Changes

A change is usually the right medicine for many areas of your life even though it may seem like the toughest solution. We have covered changing the diet and changing your thoughts, but ultimately health may require changing your environment. Where we live, where we work and who we spend that time with has an effect on our life and health. Now this can be tremendously good, and you know right now if it is or not. So you may want to start by just looking around, thinking to yourself, what gives me joy here and what makes me anxious or causes me pain. Again, expand and bring more into your life that brings joy and start minimizing or changing that that makes you weak.

There are many ways to do this as well. Start out with the realization that you have the ability to identify these areas and then make choices to change is all within your power and scope. The changes can start truly with just your awareness of wanting to work toward joy and peace in your life. The rest can be slow and subtle but all in a direction of honoring who you are and finding joy for yourself. This does not have to be at another's expense. Ultimately, when you are happy and fulfilled, so will be the folks that love and care about you - and the others, well that doesn't really matter, they will find their way too eventually.

You may start this external environment change by just re-alizing what bothers you in your own little burg. Is your home organized and clean? Is your office, your car, your gym bag, your purse? Do you have a favorite place to sit and collect your thoughts that makes you feel good? Start here to correct what may be bothering you. Check each thing. Ask do I feel good or I feel bad when I think of this item. If it doesn't feel good, change it in some way to improve your feelings about it.

Now extend this to your yard, neighborhood, town or city, and country. Once you have looked that over and observed your feelings about each, you may need to just fantasize in the short run about what would be better. Make a vision board and dream a bit about what a better situation would actually look like. Once you have done this, now look again at your associations, jobs, friends, and commitments. How do they make you feel? Be honest with yourself. Positive change can be a reality only if you become aware that things you like and don't like and the things you want to improve or remove.

Sometimes it helps to just identify it all in writing. Write a letter to yourself about it all, they way you see it today and what you would like to see in the future. Put this letter in an envelope and open it next year for a pleasant surprise. Awareness or consciousness is like magic!

An ancient practice that many use to help with their surroundings is Feng Shui. I have personally found this to be fun, inspirational, and goal-oriented. There are many approaches to this eastern principal which can be utilized in all areas of your life. You can re-stage any environment you occupy to bring a different energy to that space. I have had my homes and work spaces decorated and configured with the help of a Feng Shui consultant and have always been fascinated by the results. I have friends who have done it to find or create healthy relationships, better health, better careers, wealth and prosperity and more. It is fun and interesting and creates change, again, even just subtle change can make a major difference.

So your health and happiness is really what this chapter is about. Boldly change whatever you must to find this for yourself. Everyone that matters will be glad you did!

About the Author
DONNA LABAR

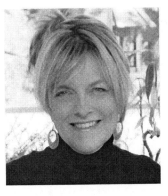

When author Donna LaBar shares her 30 years of study into nutritional healing, her eyes light up and her beauty defies her years. A lifetime resident of the rural Pennsyvania town of Tunkhannock, LaBar is sought after for healing information on cancer, diabetes, arthritis, weight loss, and more. Her gift? LaBar is a master of translating the healing power of an alkaline body into layman's terms. LaBar starts with the story of how her daughter healed from an adult form leukemia when she was a child.

LaBar receives calls for help nearly every week from individuals who do not know where else to turn. Her gentle guidance is recognized for its effectiveness, as shown in the stories she shares in her new book. She is self-taught in the field of medicinal properties of nutrition. Find out more about Donna's life work at www.DonnaLaBar.com.

Chapter 11

Freestyle Meditation

BY BERNADETTE KOZLOWSKI

Lori, an insurance account representative, was having trouble sleeping. We met at a networking dinner. When I told her I was a meditation coach, she quickly asked if I could help her sleep. Her non-stop thoughts were keeping her awake, despite her best efforts to block them out or push them away. If resistance wasn't working, I told her, then try the exact opposite and welcome those thoughts. Just don't act on them or judge them. When I saw her a month later, she was overjoyed as she had fallen asleep immediately that night and slept soundly every night since. All I had done was share one of the secrets of freestyle meditation.

By trying to block out thoughts, we stop flow. If we welcome them, but choose to do nothing about them, they will flow as they need to be. In physics, Ohm's law says that with less resistance in a wire, electricity will flow more easily. We operate as an electrical being. So, when we actively resist thoughts, we block our natural energy flows.

In meditation, brainwaves slow down, and you become deeply relaxed. So how do you access this? Another secret is that tapping into meditation is easy, since the ability to meditate is biologically wired into you for restorative balance. You just have to give yourself permission to rest, to do nothing.

My journey into Meditation

One night I was walking my dog, Dudley, in downtown Tunkhannock, PA, taking our regular route, when he insisted we go down a street we never used. Drawn to a new gift shop, I unwittingly had stumbled onto my new path. In the past 18 months, I had lost my mom and a nine-year relationship had ended painfully. I was in a funk. My heart ached and I knew I needed some guidance.

Something told me I needed to go into that store. Meeting the owner, Lori, I said I was looking for something on stress relief, maybe meditation. She didn't have anything there, but she had some personal things across the street and asked if I wouldn't mind watching the store while she ran over to get them. Only in a small town! She brought back some books and videos for me to borrow which set me on this journey. I am forever grateful.

Not long after that, my childhood friend, Kellie, invited me to a spiritual retreat in Lilydale, NY. The retreat included affirmation, energy work, inspiration, support, meditation, and breath work. During one of the breathing sessions, I went into a deep meditative state and had this incredible release of energy up and out of my body. It is hard to describe, but I had given myself permission to stop and rest and found mind, body, and spirit restored. Breathing was easier, tension was gone from my shoulders, and I was renewed.

After that weekend, my life started to open, colors were vivid once again, I had a better sense of self, and I was more present. Deciding to immerse myself in a meditation course for a week, I found myself at Kripalu in Massachusetts, learning meditation from Dr. Lorin Roche, through an immersion program. In this teacher training class, most everyone was a yoga teacher or involved in wellness centers. Here I was, the newbie, a high school biology teacher, anxious, but eager to learn about this mysterious world of meditation. I had visions of sitting in strict positions for hours, always quiet and still, learning the necessary discipline to start a practice.

Within the first hour, my preconceptions of meditation were gone. We had danced like crazy, opened our senses, and were given freedom to explore meditation. Meditation is not about hard work or discipline but great ease. We learned to be aware of our thoughts but not interested in them. I was able to slip quickly into a meditative state and was hooked!! Instead of blocking out my real world, I found my senses wide open! Time had slowed down, I was alive again!

Before leaving, I strolled down to a beautiful lake at the bottom of the hill. Instead of racing through the woods, checking my watch, and thinking about other things, I found myself meandering along the footpath, watching the green leaves move softly in the breeze, the birds flitting in the brush. I was enjoying observing the various shades of green and smelling the dampness of the woods. When I arrived at the lake and slipped into the cool water, I was transported. Best swim of my life! I can still feel the silky smoothness of the water and hear the muffled sounds as I floated on my back with my ears underwater. I was deliciously present to my world. I was in my 40s at the time and hadn't been so present since my childhood.

So, what happens between childhood and adulthood? Are you searching for a return to those days when you, as well as time, moved a little more slowly, when you had time to yourself, and were alive with a child-like wonder of the world? You knew how to access that peaceful aliveness as a child and you still know how to tap into that as an adult. You simply have to give yourself permission.

Meditation as a Healing Modalilty

Now, I can tap into the beautiful resource of meditation going from being wound up to feeling centered, often in the matter of a few minutes. Meditation has become a mini-vacation I can use anytime and anywhere, restoring me effortlessly. There are more hours in my day, the days are richer, I have a better sense of self and my boundaries, I spend less time WORKING on my problems, I can come back to center more quickly, and my intuition is much sharper. My health is greatly improved and I can go with the flow more.

My own experiences and the anecdotal evidence from my students is backed up by scientific research. After sorting through 19,000 meditation studies, Dr. Madhav Goyal and other colleagues at Johns Hopkins University published a study in 2014 which found 47 of those studies to be scientifically sound. Mindfulness meditation was found to be an effective way to reduce anxiety, depression, and pain. Dr. Goyal stated "Meditation appeared to provide as much relief from some anxiety and depression symptoms as antidepressants." His research was based on daily mindfulness meditation, actively using the senses while being non-judgmental.

Those who practice meditation have long described the mental, emotional, and physical benefits of meditation. In the first study to document actual brain changes, Harvard researchers at Massachusetts General Hospital found that meditation can cause the brain to rebuild grey matter in only 8 weeks. In the study, published in 2014, MRI images were taken before and after an 8 week study in which participants meditated for about 30 minutes per day.

Be a meditative rebel!

The key to freestyle meditation is your approach. Be a rebel on your own path. Listen to teachers that are sent your way, but decide what works and what doesn't. When starting a new group, I do an activity to illustrate this point. I tell them to follow me and pay attention to our surroundings as we walk through the church. On purpose I walk at a quick pace, down the side aisle, back up the middle aisle, and through a side door into our meeting room. There's barely enough time to stop and look at anything, but without fail, the group follows me single file, keeping pace, and follows me right back to the room. I ask them about the experience and they respond by saying they wanted to see more, they were frustrated with the pace. "This is your first lesson in meditation," I say, "I am not your leader. Do not follow me. Take your own path. As a coach, I am here to help you seek what gateway into meditation works for you."

Then I instruct them to go back to the church and explore, resting wherever they are called. People will touch the wood, smell the oils on the organ, investigate the magnificent details in the woodwork, or hug a marble pillar. Some simply sit in a pew and feel the space around them, or listen to the click of shoes on the stone floor. They return to the room, relaxed after the simple indulgence of giving into what they wanted to explore.

If you try to meditate in a way that works for someone else but not for you, you will struggle and become disheartened. Be a rebel, if it doesn't work for you try something else.

One client, Jenn, simply squirmed in a seated meditation. She loved to move, so I suggested she meditate right after her workout. She laid down right in the gym and closed her eyes for five minutes and meditated on sensations in her body. She went in deeply and easily.

GO with the FLOW

Freestyle meditation removes resistance to the natural flow of your body. So many of my clients describe wanting to stop thoughts. They intuitively say "It's impossible to stop my thoughts, can you help me?" I ask them, "If it's impossible, then why fight it?" Instead, welcome the flow of thoughts and you will be able to slide past them. A sense of relief often appears on their faces.

Our brains are made of 100 billion cells and each neuron can have up to 10,000 connections. The complexity of that web is beyond comprehension and beyond our ability to control it. So why try? In meditation, peace will come from accepting the flow, not demanding stillness.

Quality of Attention

Being with what you love allows you to be relaxed and slip past into a deep state of meditation. Put this book down for a few minutes, and ponder a time when you have been totally lost in the moment. It could be something quite ordinary or something profound.

What was it like to relive that moment? Did you feel you were in the presence of something bigger than yourself? Consider the quality of attention you experienced. You were likely engaged and embracing all that was happening. You remember it vividly. Why? Because your senses were open and engaged. You had thoughts, but you probably were paying gentle, loving attention to something, with a sense of curiosity, with love.

How do you start meditating?

Many people are aware of using a candle or a verbal mantra or the breath to meditate. In freestyle meditation, you can choose anything upon which to meditate. If it's something you love, you are much more likely to start and continue a healthy meditation practice.

God has given us this incredible human experience and wants us to embrace it by being present to it. Meditate on music, a poem, a sunset, a breeze, a baby sleeping, gratitude, peace, a feeling, the breath, movement. There are thousands of ways to meditate. You can find these in the ancient literature, at the bookstore, on You Tube, on retreat, or by simply experimenting.

Beginners are often worried about starting. *What clothes should I wear? Do I need special cushions? Can I sit on a chair instead of on the floor?* There is a palpable sense of relief when I explain that, contrary to popular belief, you can be in any position which is comfortable. You can also move, stretch, or change positions.

Don't try to empty your mind. It's not possible. Don't be afraid of not doing it right, a common theme I come across. Let everything FLOW; thoughts, emotions, feelings, and sensations. Meditation is a very rich experience, the same as your outer life. It's also expansive. Avoid using the words "focus" and "concentrate" because when you are unable to do so, you will feel like a failure, becoming frustrated. Wide open attention is so much more appealing. You can meditate on external and internal worlds. Both are textured, rich, and vast.

What will happen during/after meditation?

No matter what you meditate upon, you will alternate between rest and restlessness, as quickly as every few seconds. As long as you accept this natural cycle, you will enjoy meditation. You may be in a deep state of peace and then transition to your to do list and then back to peace again.

You may feel physically relaxed and have mental clarity. You may gain the ability to rebound more easily from setbacks. You will learn to rest in your center when there is chaos around you because you have practiced that in meditation.

Conclusion

Freestyle meditation is not cookie-cutter, but an inquiry-based approach based on a natural ability. You can explore all the different schools of meditation, but have a sense of play when exploring. If you keep in mind a rebellious attitude, a sense of curiosity, and accept FLOW in all things, you will quickly develop a healthy meditation practice!

Meditation is about spending quality time with yourself and gently paying attention to something you love. In that relaxed state, you are more likely to slide beyond into deeper states of consciousness.

Divine energy is in everyone and all things. Divine energy

is in you, and the trees and the birds and the wind, and the rain, and the mountains. When you truly open your senses to life one moment at a time, this helps you to go beyond and find the divine. Have a sense of curiosity, explore with love, accepting all that you find.

Meditation can become your anchor. You will be better able to take care of yourself physically, mentally, and spiritually. You will multi-task less often but be more efficient. When your plate gets too full, you will be able to say it can wait or no thank you. You won't have to please everyone or solve their problems. You will listen to your gut instincts more.

Give yourself permission to BE, to rest in the presence of anything YOU choose. If you feel like you are trying or working, stop and meditate later. Welcome the flow of all thoughts, emotions, and sensations in a non-repressive way. How you speak and listen to yourself in meditation are the keys to success. When you affirm all that you find during meditation, when you edit nothing, you are on the way to a healthy, vibrant way of meditating. Be ready to walk through this world differently!

About the Author

BERNADETTE KOZLOWSKI

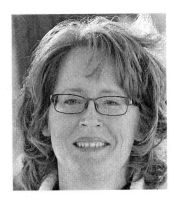 Bernadette Kozlowski is a meditation coach who helps people discover how easy it is to meditate. She especially likes working with "beginners" or people who are stuck in their practice. There really are no beginners in meditation as we are born with the ability and have used it many times, but didn't have a name for it.

As the founder of Light Your Fire Meditation, Bernadette works with private clients, small and large groups, and retreats. Programs can be customized to your needs! See how meditation can help your personal and professional life! Skype sessions are also available.

Bernadette has been in education for 25 years, teaching mostly Biology on the secondary level. This background gives her an appreciation for the science behind meditation and the ability to help each meditation student find what works for them.

She started meditating in 2010 and has seen her life change dramatically. She continues to train under Dr. Lorin Roche, an expert in instinctive meditation. She resides at Lake Carey in Tunkhannock, PA and spends her free time in the outdoors, hiking, kayaking, biking, snowshoeing, and camping.

Lightyourfiremeditation.com
Facebook: Light Your Fire Meditation with Bernadette Kozlowski
570-240-3444
Berniekoz2@frontier.com

Chapter 12

The Healing Energy of Believing

BY CATE LABARRE

"Faith is to believe what you do not see; the reward of this faith is to see what you believe." – St. Augustine

The phone call came on a cold evening in January 1995. Someone from the past called to tell me he was sick. He had just been diagnosed with hepatitis C. My heart pounded; I began to sweat; my ears rang; I could barely breathe. We were both IV drug users in the early 1970s. It was a part of my history I wanted to forget. I buried it deep, but not deep enough. In this brief phone call my shame-filled past bubbled up like toxic sludge. He was calling me, warning me, "Cate, get checked out. Don't wait to be sick." I was already sick. I had debilitating headaches, fatigue and transient joint pain – so far, the underlying cause had not been diagnosed.

I knew. It was true. I had hepatitis C. I was overwhelmed with fear. I called my nurse practitioner at home that night. I cried and shook as I shared my suspicion and my shame. She told me to come in the next day to get tested and then said, "Cate, you never told me you were an IV drug user." I responded, "Why would I volunteer something like that? Besides, you never asked!"

Denial is a normal and powerful human response to something shameful. I wished that time in my life had never happened. My own behavior so many years before horrified me. I didn't just feel that I was self-destructive and that I behaved badly, I felt like a rotten person to the depth of my being.

At that moment I hated myself as much as when I was using drugs. I was terrified that I was going to die. I did not yet know that my most important job would be to believe in myself, believe in my guidance and believe in my choices. I was setting off on the next phase of my journey to learn that the self-love and compassion I would experience from believing is the antidote to fear, dis-ease, denial, anger, addiction, shame and blame. This would become a profound healing, from the inside out.

I began to reassure myself. Hadn't I believed that I could quit doing drugs on my own? Didn't I move away, get clean and stay clean? Yes. I wanted to live. I believed that major change was ahead, that there was more for me to learn.

When I was diagnosed with hepatitis C (HCV) I had a successful practice as a massage therapist. Within months of diagnosis I had an opportunity to take a Reiki class. I didn't think that Reiki was anything special, but I decided to be open. During my attunement to this healing energy, I felt an indescribable force of love course through my body, a moment of grace. I began to calm down and trust that I could navigate my choices ahead. I became a Reiki Master Teacher and shared this gift with hundreds of college students and adults.

I recognized that my marriage was unhealthy. I believed that counseling would help and it did. It made us both realize our differences were irreconcilable and we separated. It was a painful time, and I felt terribly guilty splitting up our family. However, I believed I had made the right choice and that I could take care of my son and co-parent effectively.

I struggled with having a "clean" diet to de-stress my liver, though I believed this to be a necessary and loving act. Initially it was an outside-in job, disciplining myself and often berating myself when I failed. In addition to setting boundaries with myself, I had to set boundaries with friends. One friend told me, "You used to be much more fun at parties when you drank". I stopped taking my boring self to parties. I made new friends who supported me and my commitment to a better lifestyle.

Since there were only experimental treatments for HCV at

the time, I believed that if continued to make good choices I could survive long enough to be cured. I started working out. I lost weight. Hiking became a weekend passion and a metaphor for my life, believing with each step that I would get to the top and be a healthier, more self-loving me.

There still persisted a negative voice in my head that had been there as long as I could remember. This voice told me not to bother, because I didn't matter, I was worthless and I was unlovable. This voice caused me to return often to self-sabotaging behavior, only to create more regret and self-loathing as I would fight to regain control. This voice reminded me of my dark secrets, my shame, my pain, my past, and it would be years more before I learned to have a healthy internal dialogue with it. "Not good enough" bled into everything.

Yet all along my journey I asked for help, sometimes on my hands and knees. Show me the way. Believe it and then see it. Another moment of grace as I stumbled upon a workshop called The Shadow Process with Debbie Ford at Omega Institute. During this experiential weekend I learned that everyone has that negative "shadow" voice exactly like the one that told me "you're not important, you don't matter, don't bother". Over the next several years I trained with her as a "shadow" coach and understand the power of loving all of who I am, the parts I detested, including the addict, as well as the "I'm fine" mask I showed the world.

Several years ago my excellent gastroenterologist suggested I try a new triple-drug therapy that was proving to be about

75 percent successful in treating HCV genotype 1A, the most difficult to cure. I went for it. Nine months of excruciating treatment: hair loss, rashes, infections, exhaustion, hearing loss and eight drugs for side effects left me weak. But I believed I could get through it. I believed it would be a cure for me. I did get through it and it was NOT a cure. My belief failed me. I felt like a failure. I struggled with "why me?" "There must be a reason WHY this didn't work and I'll find out what it is!" I believed I got what I deserved! And yet another moment of grace when I dear friend sent me a book, The Gifts of Imperfection, by Dr. Brené Brown. The "shadow" that I thought I had come to know so well had a new descriptive: shame. I felt deep shame that I was not cured, that clearly this was a reflection of my lack of worthiness and the power of believing. For the next year I struggled again with believing that everything is as it should be and that it didn't matter WHY it only mattered that I love and honor myself with my beliefs, thoughts, words and actions.

I've learned that for me healing is an inside-out journey: my beliefs determine my thoughts and thoughts guide my choices and actions. I participate and collaborate. I've learned that by simply believing that there is something else for me to know or discover and my willingness to be open, miracles appear. By choosing empowering beliefs I can change the course of my life and my health. I believe in the healing power of self-acceptance and self-love. I believe in the healing power of gratitude and forgiveness. I believe I do matter, that my life is important. I awaken every day grateful, with excitement for my day and the experiences that will unfold. The virus that had been with me all those years was still there, but I was healing on so many other levels, and I believe that this is the gift.

Illness is an opportunity for you to look at your life differently. You can no longer choose how you got here; what's done is done. Whatever your healing challenge might be, it is what it is. You have one life, one body, this moment. Your illness or dis-ease is inviting you to do work on many levels, as it did me. No amount of denial, anger, blame, guilt or shame will change that. Your physical and emotional condition is not all of who you are, but it will impact you in a way that feels as though it defines you. If you feel even slightly responsible, believing that you can love yourself through it and heal may seem impossible. Making the choice to steep yourself in the reality of your current "condition" will impact your beliefs, thoughts, feelings and choices. It does not mean you are a victim. It does mean that you are free to make empowering choices from a place of love and being with "what is". You can choose what to believe.

I offer the following suggestions from my own healing experience and my exceptional training as a life coach. Know that each and every day, you can choose to listen to the fearful voice that will sabotage your self-care, or the loving voice of your believing inner healer. You have an opportunity to fully participate in your healing. You'll make mistakes and you'll have successes; you'll have bad days and you'll have great days. You'll have days when the fearful saboteur is in control and days when your believing inner healer is guiding you. You'll discover your own formula of self-love. This is your journey and you get to choose the path.

• Believe in awareness, curiosity and presence. You have only this moment. Give yourself the gift of staying present. Be curious as you practice shifting your beliefs about who you are and how you define yourself.

• Believe in healthy boundaries. Creating healthy boundaries is essential to healing. Say NO. Having to make excuses later or berating yourself for overcommitting is an energy drain. Notice when, where, how and with whom you feel uplifted or dragged down. "Energy vampires" of all kinds need to be recognized and eliminated. Notice when your own beliefs drain you, and your thoughts suck your energy. Say YES to you! Put your YOU appointments in your day planner! Massage, play, friends, fun. Believe this will give you fuel on your journey.

• Believe in acceptance and surrender. Notice if you are plagued with fear of accepting the state of your health, believing the moment you do you'll go into a downward spiral. Notice if you feel like and believe you are a victim and spend endless hours trying to figure out "why me?" Accept that you can't change the past. It is what it is. Choose to believe that there is no truth that your past determines your today and tomorrow unless you let it. Surrender doesn't mean giving up on life and being a victim. It means letting go. When you surrender, you'll see options and possibilities that are not visible in a state of denial, shame and resistance.

• Believe in forgiveness and compassion. Forgiving yourself

and others for perceived wrongs may be the biggest gift you can give yourself. Even if you are fully aware that your life-style and choices were self-destructive, it's time to give up blame. Even if others have hurt you, release yourself from this toxic energy. Forgiveness does not condone behavior, but simply helps you reclaim your vital energy and move on. You are worthy of your own compassion.

• Believe in the gift. At times when you experience a bad day, when the world seems to be crumbling down around you and you feel hopeless, ask for the gift in your experience. Let go of the expectation that life "should" be different. What do you now know because of where you are on your healing journey? Allowing today's gift into your life will diminish your distress.

• Believe in love and gratitude. Nothing can squelch fear and pain more effectively than love and gratitude. Morning and evening write down five things you're grateful for. When you find yourself in fear, take a deep breath, believe and practice gratitude. When you hurt, send love to every cell of your precious body. This will shift your perspective from pain and fear to abundance for your many blessings.

• Believe in being proactive. Research your illness and become fluent in diagnosis, treatment and prognosis. Though you may need to do much of your own inner healing work, you not meant to do it in isolation. Believe in and build a strong support network: health care professionals, therapist, alternative practitioners, counselors, coach.

• Believe in speaking your truth. Believe that it is essential to communicate clearly and truthfully from your heart. This doesn't mean dumping on others, but delivering communication that by withholding would drag you down or ultimately hurt the relationship.

• Believe in trusted confidantes. Share your health challenge with only those who are strong enough to hear the truth and those you know you can trust to hold your heart gently and with empathy. Hearing your news may make your loved one feel afraid, vulnerable and uncomfortable. Hold their hearts gently and with empathy as well.

• Believe in your higher power, grace and miracles. Perhaps nothing gets in the way of healing more than believing that you are alone. Having faith that there is a powerful, loving force outside yourself, a power bigger than your ego can comprehend, a power that will support you on your healing journey. This allows you to be humble and experience beginner's mind. "Not knowing", turning it over to your higher power, invites new insight and miracles into your life. When you fall in love with your higher power and trust your divine connection, you will know in the core of your being that you are worthy and loveable. You will trust that your choices are for your highest good.

• Believe in movement, play, creativity, laughter, joy and rest. Healing can feel like hard work. Give yourself a break. Every day! You don't need to earn joy, rest and play. Believe that you can move your body with ease. Believe in the healing power of laughter, no matter how serious your "condition". Believe in joy as a limitless commodity and not to be saved up until you are "healed".

• Believe in stillness. Allow a quiet environment. Turn off everything. Then listen to your believing inner healer, the part of you that's connected with the divine, your higher power and the healing power of the universe.

• Believe in "I"llness to "We"llness. You are unique and you are not. You are no less and no more than another. You truly are one with all that is. Believe that the most healing thing you can do for yourself is to heal in community. Ask for help. Offer help in service to others. Share your passion. Share your light.

"I believe that tomorrow is another day and I believe in miracles." – Audrey Hepburn

About the Author
CATE LaBARRE

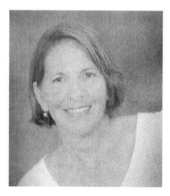

Cate's healing journey began in 1974, the day she realized that if she didn't stop using heroin she was going to die. She quit her job, packed up her apartment and left Westchester County, NY, to stay with a friend on Cape Cod to withdraw and detox. She lived and worked on the cape for about a year and returned to the metro NY area long enough to experience a brief relapse.

The synchronicity of life and her own healing beliefs saved her with a move to Upstate NY. She was caretaker of The Committee on Poetry, a 90-acre farm owned by poet Allen Ginsberg. She lived without electricity and learned how to harvest and chop wood, care for chickens, drive a tractor, manage a large vegetable garden and milk a goat. The serenity of that quiet environment has stayed with her as she has always chosen a rural setting for her home, where she feels most grounded and connected.

Cate's early undiagnosed health challenges guided to her to explore traditional medicine and non-traditional healing. She worked for physicians at a teaching hospital before pursuing her training as a NYS Licensed Massage Therapist. She expanded her bodywork practice to include craniosacral therapy and somatosynthesis, as well as Reiki. This led to further exploration of the impact of thoughts, beliefs and emotions on healing. Her training as a life coach has allowed her to take the next step in her own healing as well as supporting others on their healing journey.

Cate trained with Debbie Ford and The Ford Institute of Integrative Coaching (TFI) at JFK University. She is a Certified Master Integrative Coach & Leader. Cate is registered to complete Daring Way™ National Certification Training, July 2015, based on the research of Dr. Brené Brown. She volunteers as a mentor to coaches in training for TFI and has led support groups for women and adolescent girls. She is co-founder and co-leads the first Lean In group in her area, Saratoga Leans In. She creates and facilitates women's day and weekend retreats in the Northeast. She has also published numerous articles in health related journals. She offers private coaching, workshops and classes via phone worldwide.

Cate is passionate about supporting women who are seeking inspiration, fulfillment, optimal health and joy. She is a strong advocate of courageous living through self-compassion and caring for ourselves with the same dedication we bring to caring for those we love. She guides women to experience self-care in a unique way, recognizing that the outer "doing" of life is a direct reflection of our inner "being"; that actions and behavior are direct reflections of thoughts and beliefs. She knows that when we love and honor ourselves at the deepest level, we easily express our authentic nature, resulting in better relationships and improved health.

Cate is blessed to have a close relationship with her grown son and a thriving encore marriage. Weekends find her enjoying the outdoors with her husband hiking in the Adirondack Mountains, paddling or snow-shoeing. She and her husband live in rural community close to Saratoga Springs, NY, where they enjoy the abundance of cultural events, fun and food that this small city has to offer. Cate enjoys dancing, yoga, Pilates, painting, photography, quiet time and reading.

At the time of this writing, Cate has completed a 12-week course of Harvoni, the latest drug developed and approved for treatment of HCV, genotype 1A. Her blood work reveals normal liver function and HCV virus is undetectable.

For more:

http://CateLaBarre.com
http://TheFordInstitute.com/CateLaBarre

Chapter 13

Beautiful Broken Place

By Janet Dunn

I have been inside, upside, and turned all around for lots of my life. I was in a marriage that was abusive both mentally and physically for many years. It lasted probably more years than I care to remember. I had low self esteem issues. There were things about me I really did not like (inner demons and those low lying lizards).

I have listened to more than my share of self-sabotaging thoughts. I have been crazy with I cannot do this and then couple that with a man that said the same thing to me, over and over again.

I was frozen in this relationship. I was too afraid to change and miserable with my life. I also was stuck in my shame. Always fearful of what people would think. So I never told anyone about this situation. I did not know that my kids were sharing their stories about the family life. I knew they were afraid but never even thought they would tell anyone. Yet, no one said anything and no one confronted my husband. Why? This I do not understand.

Years went by and I half-heartedly attempted to leave. I would pack the kids in the car and drive for maybe 30 miles and then feel scared of the complete unknown. I would turn back around. I would go back to the predictable abuse and familiar uncomfortable comfortable home life. This went on for many years. My kids grew up and found their own way. They each went to college and now live many miles away.

The kids are brave and determined to live in healthy and supportive relationships. This they do with consistent attention and grace.

What about me (this small voice inside of me would say)? I tried to listen, but kept denying the voice. Maybe someday I would find a way. But still the voice never died and the voice was louder and more consistent. It was very hard not to listen. It was now at the point that it was shouting "GET OUT!"

After 35 years I left. I was in my 60s and I knew it was time. I had built the foundation for courage and I was on a mission to get my life back. I learned what it took to find my way home. I was ready to listen with my heart, pray to the angels, and ask for help. I surrendered, got on my knees more than once, and cried and asked for guidance for help. Before, I never really asked for support. I was so embarrassed and unwilling to let people know how weak I was or how weak I thought I was. I did not realize that the way to clarity and freedom was to be vulnerable. You must acknowledge the cracks. That is how the light gets in. Leonard Cohen said that years ago, and I never paid attention to such a beautiful way of noticing your life.

The process to reclaim myself came with time. I took several steps forward, took some backwards, took breaks, and went inside for answers. The years with my husband were many but I started to do what I needed to do to stay on my path.

I started a conversation with myself, listened to others, took classes, and got serious. I started to see things differently. My eyes were open and ready to see differently. I had always gotten very busy with distractions. I never would allow myself to go there. I know I was disconnected from me. My relationship with my body was nothing more than cleaning, feeding, sleeping, and clothing it. If I had been more connected, I was afraid that I would realize how much time I had wasted with this precious life.

It started with yoga training in the late 1990s. I listened with my heart. I was starting to really pay attention. I applied for a scholarship to the largest yoga institute in the country. I worked hard to make enough money to go. I even painted my neighbors trailer (it was not fun) but I had my heart set on going. Needless to say my husband told me how very selfish I was to want to do this. Selfish, I suppose it was but I had to do this. I started to even change my feelings and interpretation of the word selfish. Selfish can certainly be about taking care of yourself so that you can help others, share more, and change the vibration for the better. It took me a long time to finish the training, but I became a certified yoga instructor and I was changing. I was getting more and more connected to me, my own light, my own self, and I was getting happier. I was starting to dream about what I really wanted for myself and how this could affect others.

At this institute I also found meditation. Every day while at this center, I would take myself to the little chapel and meditate. My mind was beginning to quiet down. I was getting glimpses of soft and easy moments. I was able to see my heart's desires coming alive. I felt so much clearer when I would sit and be still for a few minutes a day. I found the connection to my body and through that I started to connect more and more to my true self. I felt like I was cracking open. Inside of that heart was ME. GRACE!

The kind of grace that is accepting of all parts of yourself and I started to know self compassion.

After that training I started teaching several yoga classes. I started really facing my own self-sabotaging thoughts but they weren't shouting at me anymore. Instead of denying them, I listened, and I talked with them. I was nurturing them and I was finding love through the process. I know that what you deny only takes on more and more of a life. I had to follow this different way. I equate them with little children that need attention. You somehow have to love them and the thoughts ease up and the voices become softer. I was offering grace to those voices, too..

When I was at Kripalu, I also found another way that soothed my soul. I was staying in a dorm situation while at my training. I roomed with 11 other women. There was a mother type for all of us (even though we were grown-up women), a whiney one, needy one, a bossy one, and this was not that different than a regular family. We were all having our buttons pushed. I knew I needed a release from my new family for awhile every day. I found dance!!! It was a class every day for one hour. It was based on the seven chakras, the rhythms of the body, and listening to the body. I felt free to move, to sway, to get deep in the hips, and I found joy. I got certified to teach dance kinetics a few years later. I found more and more joy in my life. I came back from that training and taught what I learned. It was the best therapy and I was free every time I danced.

Movement was grace.

I started to surrender more to the truth of me. I started to pay attention to what got me excited.

I learned about Feng Shui and the art of placement. I learned that the auspicious placement of things, colors, symbols, furniture, and clearing space could change your life. I went to California to study. I loved what I learned and came back with new tools for a more fulfilled life. I taught what I learned and again things changed. So much of my life was about freedom, loving my life, and finding joy.

I started getting more and more interested in nutrition. I had always eaten pretty well and had raised a lot of my own food but this was taking it to another level. I got inspired to go the Institute of Integrated Nutrition in New York. I learned how everybody is different, and each calls for different foods and diets. I learned about honoring your body with nourishing healthy food and different ways to live your life with grace. I started to teach and coach what I had learned. I learned more about listening to your body and giving it what it needs. I asked what nourishment really means. I was opening more to grace and believing that I could trust my voice and teach that to others.

I pursued another yoga teacher training certification in the Berkshires of Massachusetts. This training took me to a whole other level of yoga. I learned more yoga philosophy, yoga therapeutics, and more meditation. Breathing (pranayama) exercises clearly opened the energy of the body. It helped tremendously en terms of releasing blocks that we hold in our bodies, hearts, and minds. I simply learned yoga from a deeper perspective and first and foremost I learned how to begin by opening to grace. This theme was running through everything I was being taught. I was absorbing so much but even though the teachings were different the under current was the same, grace.

I was learning that I was here to truly get clear and connect with myself. I was also teaching what I was learning. All of the teachings, workshops, certifications, books, and classes were getting stronger within me.

I became a life coach in 2010, through Martha Beck's Institute. I wanted to learn how I could get even clearer in my life so that I could be living the life of joy and freedom. I studied how the brain works, thought work, about the body compass, and so many other tools to get free. I wanted this so I could live more in grace even with the heartache and the struggle of life. I wanted to learn the law of acceptance and to have more compassion for myself and others. I have now coached many people with so much joy and insight. I learned how to open to more grace.

I am now a retreat facilitator, a life and health coach, yoga teacher, and more than this, a person who lives her life. I am always learning to love what is.

I see my children and I am so grateful for who they are and how they have taken big chances, love their lives, and how they have learned how to be in this world and stay in grace.

In many ways I have come from a beautiful broken place but what tremendous lessons have come from there. I would not have learned what I have if I wasn't broken. I am grateful nearly every day for what created my broken-ness. I can clearly go way back to being small and remember my sadness and my confusion. What I also remember is I always pursued refuge in small places. My bedroom closet where I would spend hours just being quiet. I was just being with myself, in the playhouse way up in the Adirondack Mountains, just being with myself, being in the woods, and being in the space of spirit. I sought quiet, serenity, and peace in these places. They were like temples that I could rest in and be in. I was little and young then but some things never change. I am still looking and yearning for that quiet.

It makes life much more palatable and easier to be in. It is the place of grace. Where you can go and reconnect with self. How can we hear our small voice if we are always in noise? Please notice what is going on around you and ask yourself can I hear? I guess in a way I have been meditating since I was a young girl. Perhaps it was a different way but it was a way. I have started to remember different ways that I used to connect to spirit. When I was young I had a friend, her name was Joannie Mahogens, and she was my soul friend. I could not see her in the normal way yet I I could feel her presence. We were always together. I look back and know she was my little spirit friend my spirit guide but back then no one ever used those terms of definition.

I have been a solitary person (always preferred to be alone) not all of the time but often. My quiet times are when I get fed and I am able to connect with me. I used to think there was something wrong with me craving this time but now I know the truth. There is a part of ourselves that truly knows what is so important to us. I believe that growing up is about learning to accept who you are even the not so great parts. One of the ways to find you is by getting quiet with your Self.

So I want to offer you are some great tools to get you on the path to self discovery and back home to self.

Anne La Mont said it best: "I do not at all understand the mystery of Grace, only that it meets us where we are, never leaves us, and we are never the same because of it."

So simply allow yourself time to be with you. No distractions, close the door, turn off the external noise, get comfortable, and breathe. Try this every day even for a few moments, a few minutes, even 15 minutes. Watch your breath. When you focus on your breath your mind has a distraction and you will not be caught up in what has been referred to the "monkey mind."

As you sit and breathe you may notice thoughts but as if you were watching a blue sky with soft lovely clouds imagine the thoughts like clouds and they quietly go across the sky and disappear. This is the practice of non-attachment. You are not really focusing on the clouds just noticing them leaving the sky.

Next, take a few more moments to be with yourself in quiet. Ask yourself what your intention is for the day. This is a practice of going inside and opening to Grace. Asking for what you would like of this day or how you would like to be in this day. Set your intention is like planting a seed, planting it in your heart, and honoring and nourishing it with Grace.

This whole process is really about being more conscious of your life, your thoughts, your deeds, and creating more joy, freedom, and grace.

I believe when we wake up to our life and it's possibilities we create a life we love. When we are in that love and joy our world feels that energy and that helps others to wake up too.

So I say love your life and open to Grace in this beautiful broken place. It's your life and you have a choice to live it fully, with all its greatness and all the not-so-perfect greatness.

About the Author

JANET DUNN

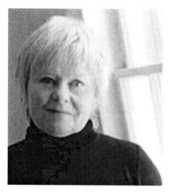

Janet has been a student of yoga for over 40 years. Her practice brought her to become a certified yoga and meditation teacher. She has found that yoga has helped guide her through her life journey. She is also a certified life coach, professional storyteller, and a retreat and workshop facilitator. Her unique style of teaching yoga comes through the weaving of story, affirmations, meditation, asanas, and through the philosophy of self-acceptance.

Janet has studied yoga for most of her life. Meditation and yoga have helped her through the passages of transitions, the easy and the challenging ones. Her intention is to live consciously and to love what is. She is a certified life coach, retreat facilitator, and health coach. She works with women who are in crisis, they are scared, need direction, and ready and willing to find the courage to love their lives.

Her greatest intention is to help you accept where you are in this moment.

Connect with Janet here:

Tao of Delicious Health http://www.taoofdelicioushealth.com
Email: TaoofHealthJLD@hotmail.com Phone: 570-242-7232

Chapter 14

Live Your Yes: The Healing Energy of Three Words

BY MEGAN WALROD

What does it mean to Live Your Yes? What is the healing energy of these three words?

These words changed my life and have become the mantra by which I live.

They have also become the name of my business (Live Your Yes, LLC) and are a guiding light in my approach to coaching clients.

How might these three words gift you with healing energy that could change your life?

How might they restore the joy and color in your life if you've been feeling gray and heavy? How might they add even more colors (and magic) to a life that you may already enjoy? How might they improve your health, relationships and business?

To answer these questions, let me first share the story of where these words came from.

Over six years ago I sat on the green leather couch in my living room, journaling, praying and crying.

"What am I not seeing?" I asked my Source. "What do I need to see?"

It was 7 a.m. My fiancé was still asleep in the other room. My morning ritual of waking up early to write had been going on for much of my adult life. My praying, crying, question-asking ritual had been going on for several weeks.

From the outside in I had it all: I was in relationship with my best friend and the man who had once been my fantasy man; we were growing a business together that was on track for making six figures in its first year; I was growing my own coaching practice; and we lived together in a small one-bedroom home with two cats in Northern California. What could be more perfect?

On the inside, I was miserable: stuck, dissatisfied and confused. This was everything I had been asking for. Why was I so unhappy? What was wrong? Why couldn't I figure out what I did want? I was going through the motions of relationship, business and life, feeling heavy and gray.

When had the color gone from my life?

I had been sharing my misery with my girlfriends for weeks, seeking understanding and guidance for what to do. On some level I knew what needed to change, I just didn't yet have the courage to speak my truth and create the radical shift that was actually required.

As I sat there on the couch that morning, something was different. Recently I'd been struggling with some mysterious health issues. I was literally getting sick from my misery. I was finally ready to see what I had been hiding from in my depression.

"Universe, what is going on?" I implored. *"Talk to me. Tell me. Help me see."*

That's when I heard, in a voice that was not really a voice but a vivid awareness that was so real it was undeniable, *"You've been living your maybe."*

Tears poured down my cheeks at receiving a message from the beyond that reverberated through me as truth: I had been hiding out in a safe harbor.

This life I had so excitedly built from scratch after the destruction of my divorce was no longer a match for me. My heart wasn't fully in any of it. Not the relationship or our shared business. And how could my own coaching business be enjoyable or successful when my heart wasn't in my life?

"So what do I do?" I asked, begging for more answers.

That's when I received the gift that would change my life forever.

Three words surged up from my belly to my heart: **Live Your Yes.**

My body shook with receiving this message. Although I didn't know what living my Yes looked like, I felt the energy of these three words. I felt the healing they offered as they invited me to live a life with my heart fully participating in (and guiding) my choices.

Live Your Yes. Live Your Yes. Live Your Yes.

These three words became my mantra. The heavy cloud I'd been walking around in cleared. I knew what needed to be done: in order to Live My Yes I needed to release the ties that held me in the safe harbor.

A few days after my morning epiphany I had a dream of a rainbow-colored ferris wheel. In the dream some men drove off with my wallet: in it was my license – my "identity." As I stood there on the side of the road I looked up and saw the bright colors of a painted wheel spinning in the sky.

I knew, in that sweet unshakeable way you know things, that I needed to move to Santa Cruz (it was the only place around that had a Ferris wheel), that I would be ok, and that I was getting the chance to re-create my life and who I knew myself to be – in Technicolor!

With as much grace as I could muster, I ended my relationship and our business partnership. I was scared and excited. I didn't know what was going to happen. I just knew this:

I was no longer willing to stay in a maybe life when I knew a Yes life was possible.

And so the adventure began of Living My Yes, and inspiring others to do the same.

Now, six years later, I live a Yes life. My business is thriving. I work with global thought leaders and women entrepreneurs around the world. I travel to exotic places like Bali, Costa Rica, Hawaii, Mexico and beyond. I am in a new relationship with an Enjoyable Other and experience more fun and pleasure than ever before.

The mysterious health issues I once had have dissolved. I have more energy and vitality. I flow through my days writing, coaching, laughing and creating. I still wake up early and write yet now I am filled with joy and gratitude for the life I live.

This is not a static life. It is a very dynamic one that invites me to continuously ask:

"Am I living my yes?"

"What brings me most alive?"

"Am I choosing that which lights me up?"

As I discovered so many years ago, what can start off feeling like the right fit or a great life can become a mismatch and a good life. I no longer settle for or accept a good life. I am continuously creating a great life, a life based on my Yes.

Woven into the fabric of a Yes life is contentment and gratitude for what is. There is not a sense of anything missing. There is excitement for what else I might create and experience as I live my yes.

And as I share with my clients: when we Live Our Yes, we create greater success for everyone. When we are Living Our Yes, our joy, our inspiration, we inspire others to live their own Yes.

Because truly, doesn't living a no or a maybe life breed discontent, disharmony and dis-ease?

What kind of world might we create together when we are all living our yes?

This is the world I am most committed to choosing, creating and inspiring.

Does creating a Yes life resonate with you?

If so, I'd like to share with you the eight steps I took to Live My Yes. May they guide you in your journey of Living Your Yes, so you, too, experience greater joy and harmony.

Step 1: Get Honest With Yourself

Take a look in the mirror and ask yourself: "Am I living a no life? A maybe life? Or a yes life?"

Signs you are living a NO life:

- You are dissatisfied, stuck and miserable.

- You feel stopped by a healing crisis or other circumstance that feels insurmountable.

Signs you are living a MAYBE life:

- You are uncertain, bored or depressed.

- You are wondering, "Where do I go from here?" and "Is this all there is?"

Signs you are living a YES life:

- You are happy, grateful and inspired.

- You flow in the abundance of all that you create. Your life is full of magic and possibilities.

Step 2: Be Willing To See Yourself

Deep down I knew what changes I needed to create in my life to move towards greater happiness and satisfaction. Yet I was afraid. I had built my life around a relationship and questioned my ability to be ok on my own.

It took being willing to see what I had been hiding from

in my depression to receive the healing message from my Source, "Live Your Yes."

You may be hiding what you know in a cloud of depression or uncertainty, just like I was. Are you now willing to see and know what you know?

Step 3: Trust Your Knowing

If you are living a no life or a maybe life, ask yourself, *"What do I know about this?"*

Be willing to not know the answers for a while. Be open to how the 'answers' come. They may not come like mine did. One morning you may wake up and just know what you need to do. Or another option may become so obvious to you that was never apparent before.

Trust what you know. Trust that you know more about your situation than you've been willing to see.

Step 4: Speak Your Truth

What changes are required for you to Live Your Yes?

Be willing to courageously speak your truth to yourself and to the necessary people in your life in order to get into greater harmony with your Yes.

In my journey of Living My Yes I realized that I would rather disappoint another than disappoint myself. I saw it was time to show up for myself in a big way even if that meant not doing or being what someone else expected of me.

When you speak your truth you may "disappoint" another and yet – at what cost would it be to choose another over yourself?

Step 5: Listen To Your Heart

The energy of Live Your Yes began to inhabit my heart. These words became an invitation to me to inhabit my heart and live from my desire and joy.

What lit me up? What called to me? At first I didn't know – I just knew what was pulling at me, keeping me tied to my maybe life. Once I said No to my relationship and our shared business, I released myself from the safe harbor and set sail for what lay beyond.

From that moment on, whenever I was exploring options for something, I tuned into my heart: which path lit me up the most?

I began to discover what I felt in my body when I was a strong Yes to something: my chest opened and I felt a lot of bubbly lightness inside. I'd often smile and spontaneously clap. These became cues for me to know something was a Yes.

Anything other than this: a heavy feeling, a constriction in my chest, became signals of my No.

Play with this yourself: what are the cues you receive from your body and beyond for what is your Yes? And what are the cues for your No?

Now: trust your knowing (Step 3) and choose your yes.

This is the only way to Live Your Yes! Listen and act on your Yes.

Step 6: Be Willing To Let It All Go

What had once been my dream life became my maybe life. I had to be willing to let it all go to create a new life based on my Yes.

Your Yes life one day can become a Maybe life the next day. Sometimes it happens overnight, other times it occurs gradually. Yet you'll know.

When you're willing to let it all go and create a new life, you don't ever need to worry about regrets or becoming stuck in a life that no longer lights you up.

Are you willing to let it all go?

Step 7: Acknowledge The Creator That You Are

It took me a while, yet I finally saw how I was playing the victim in my life: first after my divorce and then again during those months of feeling stuck. I was upset with my fiancé. I was upset with everything outside of me. I was waiting for something to change, for someone else to 'save' me.

When I received the healing message, Live Your Yes, I realized the only one who could change my life was me. No more waiting. No more looking outside myself for rescue. I now had an inner compass to guide me: my Yes.

When I turned inwards and listened to my heart, everything

began to change. I gained clarity on what wasn't working for me and what I desired, courage to speak my truth, and confidence to let go of everything in order to create my Yes life.

Now you have an inner compass to guide you in living your Yes life.

The healing energy of these words is powerful: when you choose to Live Your Yes you move beyond dissatisfaction, disharmony and dis-ease and create soul satisfaction, harmony and ease.

The healing energy of Live Your Yes is both inclusive and expansive: as you Live Your Yes, you send out ripples of healing energy inviting others to Live Their Yes.

What kind of world might you create for yourself when you choose to live your Yes?

What kind of world might we create together when we are all living our Yes?

About the Author

MEGAN WALROD

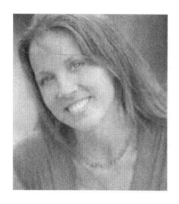

Megan Walrod, M.A., Founder of Live Your Yes, LLC, is a coach, writer, speaker, and muse. She supports women entrepreneurs to craft magnetic marketing messages that attract more Yeses from their ideal clients.

Megan has coached hundreds of entrepreneurs, supporting them to grow their business to six figures and beyond while living their purpose. She was one of the lead coaches, trainers and copywriters for a premier seven-figure company in the marketing industry. Before that, she was a consultant for a Global Fortune 500 Company, writing communications and delivering trainings for an international audience.

She received a Master's degree in Organization Development (from Bowling Green State University in Ohio) and one in Transpersonal Counseling Psychology (from Naropa University in Colorado). Her love of learning is surpassed only by her love of words and using them to inspire and empower.

Megan encourages her clients to Live Your Yes, knowing that when we live an inspired life, we are more magnetic and create greater success for everyone. Megan encourages her clients to Live Your Yes, knowing that when we live an inspired life, we are more magnetic and create greater success for everyone. To find out more about Megan (and sign up for her free gift), visit her website : www.MeganWalrod.com.

Chapter 15

A Life Beyond
the Imagined

By Stephanie Richardson

For the first 27 years of my life, I struggled with depression. Loneliness was as familiar as sunrise and the deep longing for purpose, meaning and success seemed like a permanent part of my daily life. I tried modality after modality, seeking change. The library of books I read on everything from religion to relationships helped only marginally to improve what I began to wonder might be a permanent state of dissatisfaction.

Other people seemed to have this living thing down to a science. Daily life didn't seem to bore them and routine seemed to be a comfort, even if they didn't like it. I envied what looked like ease with day to day living... but I was antsy.

I began to pursue bigger dreams... and still felt stuck.

And then I discovered something really different. I came across something called Access Consciousness®. I discovered a plethora of tools that have been a dynamic contribution to changing the very foundation of what had kept me stuck in pain in my life. The premise is simple. What if you were an infinite being? What if all things are changeable? What if you have choice? And... What if asking questions any time you come to a conclusion opens the door to possibilities you may have never imagined were possible?

How does this apply to healing? What if everything was just a choice... even healing and happiness? It's a simple concept. And a radical one.

One of the things I know is that when you are in a place of hurting or depression or dis-ease it can feel like an impossible reach to believe that you are whole, that you are not broken, that your body or your mind or your heart is not against you. But what if our bodies are not the problem? What if our bodies actually hold a key to healing, to health, and to a different way of being in the world? What if much of the discomfort, the hurting, the dis-ease, or the pain, actually wells up as information that your body is attempting to give you. What if that information was the information that you have been asking for that you thought would never show up? What if, everything that appears to be broken or dis-eased is actually a road map to your awareness – to the part of you that knows exactly how to heal?

As a friend of mine says, "It never shows up the way that you think it will!"

What if dis-ease is just a sign-post pointing to what you've been asking for but have not yet chosen?

What if you and your body truly know what it takes to heal?

What if the changes you would like to make are easier than you've ever imagined?

So, just for the duration of this chapter I'd like to ask you to put aside everything you've been told... Absolutely everything...about health, about healing, about your body, your emotional well being... all of it... all the facts, figures, the lessons, and all the teachers, gurus, and experts.

For the next five minutes, what if you and your body were the experts of what was true for you? Let's just see what would happen if you begin to really get the sense of what resonates as true for you. What if you could trust that sense, that awareness, to guide you to what you and your body require?

As you change, as your body changes, as your life changes, you may find that what you require will change too... the food that nourishes you today may not nourish you in the same way tomorrow... the routine that nourished you today may not nourish you tomorrow... the people that may nourish you today may not nourish you tomorrow.

What do you do with the things that are not nourishing to you? Nothing. It's actually easy. Changing what isn't working doesn't require boundaries or plans or strict diets. It doesn't require getting rid of those things or taking up new things in any specific way. What it does require is a completely different skill. Instead of creating new rule sets for yourself to follow, what if you cultivated the willingness to ask questions? "What would I like to choose? Would I like to choose this for me today? Yes? No?"

Just take what works for you and leave the rest... and in the next 10 seconds and the 10 seconds after that... what if what you knew was like quick sand... what if what you knew was like an ever-changing stream of information?

How do you access that information if you never hold onto any of it? If you've ever been around a curious child with non-stop questions... it's like that!

When you begin to ask questions, it begins to create a whole new level of freedom. You never have to dump the things that are not nourishing for you today. You can just ask, "Would I like to choose this today? Will this begin to create the life, the health, the body that I would truly like to have?"

The first time I remember using this tool was when I was in my early 20s. At that point in my life I spent a lot of time VERY depressed. I had been on and off depression medication with varied results. One medication made my head tingle and made me really angry all the time, another left me so tired that I could hardly sit in a chair without falling asleep, and one, the least offensive, just made everything... sort of... ok. I didn't want to have a life that was just... sort of... ok... so I ventured off medication (a discussion for another time). I was doing well and feeling good! I exercised and ate well and made friends. And then... I had that dreaded moment... the feeling of the kind of loneliness that is unwavering even in the presence of friends . And then, that unsquelchable darkness of what I nicknamed, "the nothing" began to loom on the horizon... "Oh no..." I thought, "Here we go again..."

Then, I stopped myself.

I still remember. I was in my car on the way to a friend's house. I was literally sitting at a stop sign when a question popped into my head, "Are you really willing to be happy?"

Me: "Pfft! Of course I'm willing to be happy... who wouldn't want to be happy?"

The question: "Really look at this! Are you REALLY willing to be happy?"

Me: "I don't want to look at this! What if my answer is, 'No'? Will I have to stay depressed forever?"

The question: "....?"

Me: "Ugh! If I'm not willing to be brutally honest with myself about this, who will I be honest with? And what will happen? If I'm not honest now, I won't have a chance... fine."

I sat there and imagined actually being happy... REALLY happy. I was surprised what I saw. In my imagination, being happy wasn't pleasant at all! Being happy was EXHAUST-ING!!!! It took WAY too much energy to be happy... It made me want to take a nap.

Me: "Oh my goodness! NO. I'm not actually willing to be happy! That's so weird! hahahahaha...."

Then, a funny thing happened. In those few minutes of asking questions and being willing to look at whatever came up, no matter what it looked like, even when I thought it might mean I had to stay depressed forever, the loneliness lifted. The clouds of depression looming on the horizon disappeared, and I started to laugh with the most sincere joy I'd had in years (and years)!

What!? By asking a couple of questions, and by admitting I wasn't willing to be happy, I'm happy? How is that possible?

The depression had been a huge sign pointing to a decision that I had made, at some point, that happiness required too much energy, that being depressed was easier than being happy. Where that belief came from wasn't important. It could have been someone else's point of view that I had bought or accepted as true, it could have been something I saw and resisted. Whatever the reason, the "why" didn't hold the key. Acknowledging that I had lived based on the point of view that happiness was exhausting, however, gave me the key to a doorway that I hadn't known existed until I asked the question... "Am I truly willing to change this?"

When you find that you are hurting emotionally, physically, or otherwise, would you be willing to look at where it is a signpost for something else? A signpost for where the life that you could choose and the life you are actually choosing are not lining up... a place where you know you can choose something greater and have decided that it isn't possible.

What if the life you know deep down should be possible is actually possible? Would you be willing to consider the possibility that you could change one tenth of a hundredth of a percent today?

Would you be willing to look at one of the decisions that you have made along the way that is creating the dis-ease or the lack of ease that's showing up for you now?

How do you begin to untangle the decisions and judgments that are controlling your life? Just begin to ask! Actually, let's break it down...

TOOL BOX:

Step 1: Get a sense of one thing that you would like to heal in your life... Just get a sense of one thing. You may have one thing that pops up for you and then another thing pops in with something like, "Yeah but I'm more important... you should want to heal me first, I'm a bigger deal than that other thing... that other thing is silly/shallow/lame/so small compared to this." If that happens for you, would you be willing to take the first thing that popped up and work with it? No matter how small, it may seem... no matter how it compares with anything else...

Now that you have that thing...

Step 2: What is this? When you have a sense of that one thing that you would like to change, you may discover that you have all sorts of definitions around it. If you've done any work with a therapist or with friends or mulled over it with some form of scrutiny, you may have given this thing some definitions already. Take everything that you think you know about this thing and put it aside... you can have it back later if you'd like... for now, let all of those definitions go. A definition may be, "I have an unhealthy attachment to my ex-girlfriend" or "There's too much chaos in my life. I need to get grounded." or it could be a diagnosis, "I have bipolar disorder." It could even be something as seemingly solid as, "I have stage 4 cancer." What we want to do is drop all the definitions and then just ask, "Hey... what is this?"

When you ask, it's not actually to get a cognitive answer. We usually have a LOT of those already. If we could use our minds to move beyond our problems, wouldn't we be free already? So we're not looking for more definitions or cognitive points of view... what we're doing is actually being willing to really just be with whatever the energy of this "thing" is without the struggling, without the fighting without the definitions or the figuring it out. Sometimes we're so busy fighting those things that we don't actually just sit with them and ask "Hey... so what's actually going on here?"

Unfortunately the rest of this step doesn't have any real clear way to go about it. You just ask the thing you want to change, "Hi... what is this?" and really just get a sense of it. Does the sense show up within your body? Does it show up outside of your body? Does it show up behind you under you to your left or right? Does it encompass you? Does being with it in this way begin to change it at all?

If what I'm saying seems confusing, you can just imagine sitting on a park bench next to the thing you'd like to be different. Sit next to it as if it was someone you thought was interesting but didn't really know. You ask the same way you'd say, "Hi, who are you? What brings you here?" You ask with a kind curiosity and see what you become aware of.

Step 3: Would I be willing to change this?

Actually ask yourself, "Am I actually willing to change this?" This is the part where the obvious answer is, "Of course!" But really be with it. If this changed, what else in your life would change? What else would have to change?

Imagine that what you've asked to heal is already healed. Is it a relief? Is it a stress? What comes up?

Things to consider: Does this thing give you an excuse to not go to work? Does it give you a reason to not let other people get close to you? Does it give you a way to ask for the care or the love or the touch that you would like to have in your life? Does it get you the support you crave? Does it allow you to say no? Does it allow you to be right? Does it allow you to get even? Does it bring in money? Does it keep you from having too much money?

Sometimes what comes up is really sneaky. If you've been under-employed and you say you'd really like to have a great job... you may imagine that you now have the job you've been asking for. For a split second you're relieved until... the thought pops up, "Oh! Then I have to start paying back my student loans!" Or if you would really like to heal from cancer and you imagine it being gone only to realize that it would mean you have to do something different with a relationship that isn't working.

If you run into any of these kinds of thoughts you can run this whole process on them as well... What is this? Am I willing to change it? How do I change it?

Step 4: How do I change this?

If you find that you are willing to actually have this thing change, you can begin to ask, "What would it take to change this? What energy can I be that would change this? What consciousness can I be that would change this? What space can I be that will change this?"

Whether you get a cognitive answer or not is not important. What happens when you begin to ask is that you begin to receive what you are asking for. How does that information show up? It shows up in a million different ways. You may have the desire to turn on the radio and hear someone talking about something you've been wanting more information about... you may step onto an elevator and hear people talking about a supplement or a book or a place that you just know you need to check out. You may have a craving to wear certain colors or eat certain food...

What if this is actually the adventure of healing and the adventure of creating a vibrant thriving life...? Are you ready for the adventure?

About the Author

STEPHANIE RICHARDSON

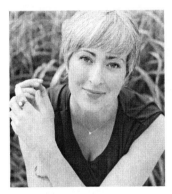

For years Stephanie Richardson longed to have purpose more than almost anything else. She wanted to know that she was contributing to the world. She wanted to be everything she could be and show up dynamically, expressively, and even inspirationally! Unknowingly, that WANT of a purpose became her platform.

The pursuit of purpose can easily become the primary use of person's time and energy. The challenge that Stephanie discovered in herself is that the pursuit of purpose never created the awareness required to take action toward a different target. For Stephanie it seemed to always loop back into requiring more purpose and more seeking of more purpose.

When Stephanie discovered the tools of Access Consciousness, she began to apply a different set of tools to her daily life, the foundation she had built on want and lack began to shift. She discovered that she could ask questions and take action without judging her purpose or her plan first. When she did those two things, the larger desires that she had began to unfold without all of the angst, struggle, and worry.

When angst, struggle and worry, however subtle, aren't working, what else can we choose? We've all wanted something greater for ourselves or for the world... what can we be or ask today that would begin to create that as a possibility right away?

Stephanie Richardson travels the world as an artist, a photographer and a Facilitator of Access Consciousness, facilitating individual sessions and group classes. For more information and free tips on the blog, you can go to www.StephanieRichardson.com.

Can't wait for more? You can listen to her radio show, The Good Girl's Guide to Being Wrong (and happy) with Co-Host Heather Smith at http://www.guidetobeingwrong.com.

Chapter 16

Are You Getting Younger Each Day?

By Pat Duran

If you didn't think you would age, would you? Thought provoking, eh? That's a question posed by Gary Douglas, the founder of Access Consciousness®. It turns out there is a lot of evidence pointing to how much our thinking, our conclusions, our points of view about growing older influence how we move through this space.

My Telling Story

I've never thought much about my age. There've been times when I actually had to do the math to figure out how old I was. Then I turned 65. Yikes! *A Senior Citizen!* How is that possible? I haven't even accepted that I was middle age! I started seeing reminders of my age everywhere. Medicare and the monthly bills. Senior discounts almost everywhere.

Friends retiring. And what did I do? I created sciatica. I wasn't able to do much work for a few months. I wallowed in it. Then I realized that my age was just a number and, other than the sciatica, I still felt like I was in my 40s. I started making different choices. I explored many areas for healing and each contributed in its own way. Still I think that shifting my attitude was the main thing that helped. My doctor had plans to talk me into getting a cortisone injection and I surprised him with my report of no more symptoms. He was amazed that it had healed so quickly. Not your average 65-year-old here!

Our Culture's View on Aging

Did you ever celebrate a milestone birthday and have people give you cards and gifts about being "over the hill" or even coffin and grim reaper jokes because you're so close to death now? Have you bought into this reality's notions about aging? Even the term "aging" itself has such meaning for people. You never ask how a child is aging – they're growing up or growing older. What would it be like if we just grew older (I'm not sure I'll ever grow up!) instead of aging?

And what if you considered all of those cultural and societal notions about aging to be just an interesting point of view? What if every time you heard someone say something about aging, you thought "interesting point of view"? And what if you catch yourself with one of those thoughts and say "interesting point of view I have that point of view"?

Did you know that people-over-age-90 is the fastest growing segment of our population? And that by 2030 there will be over 800,000 people over 100? What would it take for us to shift our attitudes about growing older by then? Or right away?

Science Supports the Impact of Beliefs

The noted physician, author and women's expert, Christiane Northrup, recently did a special for PBS called Glorious Women Never Age and she emphasized the importance of our language and our beliefs. In Access Consciousness®, the conversation is about Points of View, which are subject to change vs. beliefs that usually are pretty firm. What if all the things you've held as beliefs were just interesting points of view? Does that feel light to you? Does that assist in the possibility of changing them? Would you be willing to consider other possibilities? Dr. Northrup shared a number of studies that showed that our points of view created our reality more than anything physical, including our genes!

Five Keys to Thriving while Growing Older

KEY #1: Choose Your Words

The words we use have meaning. We spoke above about "aging" and a phrase like "over the hill". There are so many other words and phrases common in our vocabulary. Do you ever say "I'm having a senior moment"? Here's an interesting factoid: you are getting 250 times more information in one day than a person got in an entire year in 1900. Our biology simply hasn't caught up.

How about the term "anti-aging"? Any time we resist something we solidify it and give it strength. So let's not be anti anything! Let's be for growing older with joy and pleasure and vibrancy.

Retirement? Is that another word for "no longer useful" or "getting old and decrepit"? I don't imagine I'll ever retire, especially with meaning like that ascribed to the term.

Have you heard about someone who died soon after retirement? I knew a woman who had a successful career and had not had children. So much of her identity was wrapped up in her work that she didn't know who she was after she retired. She missed making a contribution and feeling appreciated. She thought she was "supposed to" take it easy and relax and do leisure activities. But that got old after a few months and, because of the meaning she ascribed to "retirement" and her beliefs about it (see next section on beliefs), she went downhill quickly.

This has become such an issue in our culture that there is even an entire coaching certification program called "Too Young To Retire". It's one of the many coaching certifications I earned after leaving my corporate job. It helps people who have retired from full-time employment consider other options, like consulting, volunteering, traveling, etc.

On the other hand, my friend Charlotte retired early last year, and she is treating it as the opportunity to do so many things she didn't have time to do when she was working. She's taking classes, volunteering, traveling, renovating her family's cabin, spending more time with friends. She's even looking for a new puppy! Her life is rich and her health is great!

Me? I'm lucky that the work I do now is something I can continue to do until the day I die. I enjoy it enough that I suspect I will do just that!

KEY #2: Shift Your Point of View

One longitudinal study found that people who believed that growing older was associated with something positive lived on average 7.5 years longer. The study was controlled for cholesterol, blood pressure, heart disease, smoking, obesity and lack of activity. *The belief itself* was more potent than any of those!

Do you ever say "I'm too old to do that!" or "At my age, what do you expect?" Or do you take in it when someone says these things to you? Would you be willing to release those conclusions? What if being older actually opened up new and different possibilities for you based on the wisdom you have?

A study of centenarians across seven continents found many things they all had in common. The centenarians were all future-oriented. They'd talk about things they were going to do in three years. They didn't preface it with "if I'm still around then".

I'll tell a tale about myself. I went through early menopause in my early 40s. I had been taking a birth control pill that stopped my periods. When I went off it, the periods never came back and, after several months, my doctor determined that I was in menopause. I started getting hot flashes even though I hadn't had a single symptom until the doctor declared me in menopause. That's the strength of some of these beliefs. What have you decided menopause must be like that you'd be willing to release now?

It would have been different if I had known about Access Consciousness® then. Access has so many useful tools – two in particular would have been very handy. Saying **"interesting point of view"** to myself every time someone told me about menopause symptoms would have been useful! The other tool is based on how empathic we are. We pick up so much from other people – our parents and siblings, friends, colleagues, even the person next to us on line at the store.

The second tool is **"Who does that belong to?"** When you have a thought, feeling or emotion that isn't working for you, ask that and if it lightens up, then it's not yours! And you can *Return to Sender with Consciousness Attached.* Try that for a few days and see how your life changes!

Some people feel that growing older lessens their value and makes them invisible. What if you reframed it as increasing your wisdom and value and becoming a stealth force of potency?

Another study put men age 70 to 85 in a closed environment, surrounded by artifacts of the 50s. They had old TVs and appliances, TV shows and magazines from the 50s, family photos from that time. They were instructed to act as if they were in the prime of their life – not reminisce but act "as if". After only two weeks, they came out looking 10 years younger with improved vision, hearing, lung function and muscle mass.

Would you be willing to give up the judgments and conclusions you have about what you have to look like, feel like, and be like as you get older? Drop the barriers and open to possibilities?

Dr. Northrup had a funny story about being asked her age. Her response was "My biological age is 35 and getting younger. My wisdom age is around 300!" LOL. I'll have what she's having! By the way, she never takes the senior discount and she keeps her chronological age top secret.

KEY #3: Nurture Your Body and Make It Your Ally

How many judgments of your body do you have? The wrinkles, the sagging, less stamina, more aches and pains, slower healing, maybe extra pounds. Would you be willing to let go of those and start appreciating your body for all it does for you? How about whenever you catch yourself judging your body, you take a moment and acknowledge three things about your body that you are grateful for? For me, it's often about being able to see, hear, feel, and smell the beauty of nature. Tasting great food and wine. Being able to walk wherever I desire to go. Hearing the sound of laughter.

So many things I couldn't do without my dear sweet body.

Here's a suggestion. Start each day asking your body "Body, what can I do today to nurture you?" I sometimes become aware that my body wants to go for a walk, or luxuriate in the Jacuzzi, or have a glass of champagne, or simply to rest. You may become aware of something your body desires as soon as you ask, or an hour later or even days later. Getting an answer isn't even that important. It's asking the question and staying in the question that opens up possibilities. It also begins to establish a collaborative relationship with your body.

You can also ask your body what it wants to wear. And when and what it wants to eat. How it wants to move. How often do we have an exercise ritual and we stick to it even when our body isn't up for it? The word "exercise" has some less-than-useful meaning. Doesn't "movement" sound much nicer?

I have a client who has lots of pain in his body yet he continues to ride his bike 30 to 40 miles at a time. His body is telling him it wants something different and he's not willing to listen. He keeps overriding his body. How many times has your body given you cues that you couldn't hear?

In the centenarians study mentioned earlier, one of the big things they had in common was **mindful rituals of pleasure**. The ritual itself would vary but they all seemed to have something that gave them great pleasure – a cigar, a glass of whiskey, etc. They savored those things.

I've started using a beautiful wine glass for my water that I sip throughout the day. It gives me pleasure and I find I'm drinking more water as a result. I happen to be single at the moment and, for a while, I wouldn't sit outside with a cocktail by myself. Then I realized how much I enjoy sitting there looking at the beautiful view of the foothills while savoring a glass of champagne. I think "savor" may be my new favorite word.

As I write this, I'm savoring the afternoon I just spent trading body processes with some clients and introducing someone to the Bars®, the fundamental body process in Access. It was a beautiful day so we played outside. We did the body work and some verbal clearings, and enjoyed snacks and good conversation. How did I get so lucky? And when I finish tonight's writing, I'm jumping in the jacuzzi.

What would it take for you to savor your body and your life?

KEY #4: Be Grateful

In the late 1990s I read about gratitude journals in the book *Simple Abundance.* I've been writing mine ever since. At night before I go to bed, I write down at least five things I'm grateful for. Some days it's not easy and I grasp for some old standards like my dogs and having my eyesight and the air I breathe. Even the toughest day of my life – the day my Mom died – I was able to come up with lots of things I was grateful for. I was grateful to have her for my Mom in the first place. All the fun times we had. All she taught me. I actually had a very long list that night. But most times I wind up with more than five very quickly. And then I feel better and I drift off to sleep with that yummy gratitude feeling.

I got to wondering about gratitude and longevity and did some googling. The results are pretty spectacular. Keeping a gratitude journal caused study participants to report fewer physical symptoms, less pain, more and better quality sleep, lower depressive symptoms, lower blood pressure, more time exercising, greater vitality and energy. Wow! Gratitude created improvements in health, emotions, personality, social interactions, and even career! All of these contribute to greater happiness. How does it get any better than that? I found a great article at http://happierhuman. com/benefits-of-gratitude/.

What are you grateful for today? Are you willing to be the space of gratitude?

KEY #5: Choose Who You Hang Around With

For several years now we've been hearing that our income tends to be about the average of the five people we hang around with the most. Well, it appears there is something similar about our health and longevity.

I remember the first year after my parents retired and moved to Florida. They weren't sure where they wanted to live so they just rented an apartment in Pompano Beach. They were surrounded by a variety of people – some older, many young with children. They befriended one family with two little girls and Mom quickly became their surrogate grandma. When I visited them, they were both happy and vibrant. After the first year they chose to buy a condo in a senior community (55+ and no kids). Everything changed then. Next time I visited and sat around the community pool with their friends, it seemed there was almost a competition to see whose illness was the worst. They just sat there and talked about all their ailments. And when they tired of that, they talked about some injustice they felt had been perpetrated on them.

Then their friends started dying. Dad went downhill quickly.

What does your community of friends talk about? What are their beliefs? Do they play the "Woe is me" game or do they know that they always have a choice in how they respond to things. Better yet, do they know they can create something different?

I think Mom survived a lot longer partly because she was 10 years younger and partly because she stayed active with various entrepreneurial ventures. She had been a book-keeper in New York and she started keeping books for the family she had befriended who also owned a pharmacy. She worked part-time at the pharmacy. She started helping the "old folks" with their finances – paying bills, filing insurance claims and taxes. I remember laughing at her talking about the "old folks" when she was 80 herself. Now I recognize that attitude was what kept her young.

Guess what the centenarians said? They don't like to be around old people!

Do you want to know what makes women happy and healthy? Their girlfriends! And what makes men happy and healthy? The women in their lives. It seems pretty clear. If you'd like to be happy and healthy, get some good women in your life!

Pets are great for this too. I know the animals who live with me add so much to my life and to my clients. They climb on my massage table when I'm doing body work and they always seem to know where to sit to contribute to that person. It's fairly often that we hear of a therapy dog working wonders with kids or patients in hospitals or elder care facilities. Animals are great healers. They do their best to heal their people, often by taking on illnesses themselves. No wonder studies show that people with pets live longer.

In Closing

What do you choose? It's really up to you how you grow older. How about we grow older together in gratitude for our bodies and our lives, contributing to the people we care for and our planet up until the day we leave our bodies? What are the infinite possibilities?

About the Author

PAT DURAN

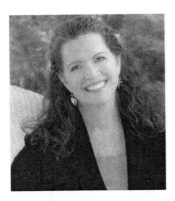

Pat Duran's gift is facilitating people to recognize their own wisdom and their own power. She is an intuitive healer and teacher, an Access Consciousness® Certified Facilitator, Bars and Body Process Facilitator, life coach, and NLP Health-certified Master Practitioner. Her whole life she has been on the leading edge, introducing ideas and practices that change people's business and personal lives. From software engineering practices in her early business career, to rapid decision making and innovative group facilitation and consulting methods, to coaching methods, to mediumship, and now to many different energy healing modalities. She loves introducing a new idea and watching the sparkle in people's eyes as they recognize all the ways it applies to their lives. She credits her love of variety and learning with contributing to her youth!

For over 30 years Pat has been guiding clients to discover what they know and who they are. At Hewlett-Packard she used to joke that her job as a consultant/coach was to work herself out of a job! She specializes is getting people their outcomes quickly and uncovering hidden talents and abilities in the process. She has an amazing ability to hone into the core of an issue and clear it.

You can contact Pat for classes and private sessions at www.AccessThe-Possibilities.com.

Chapter 17

The Inside Story

By Robyn M James

"What lies behind us and what lies before us are tiny matters compared to what lies within us." – Ralph Waldo Emerson

Sophia

I leaned over her, my face completely above hers. I looked at her as she lay anesthetised on the operating table. Aloud, I spoke to her clearly and directly. "Hello Sophia. My name is Robyn and with your permission I am going to perform surgery on you to remove your brain tumour." I received her slightly puzzled permission, as if she wanted to furrow her brow at me. I responded by gesturing towards the hospital's surgeons already at work around her and offered her verbal reassurance that she was in good hands. She relaxed. This was to be my first energetic scrub in. It would be profoundly transformative.

When I first heard about Sophia's tumour, I instinctively wanted to help – well that's really the only reason we ever hear these stories! But there was a sense of urgency for me – I wanted to meet her, to talk with her. I wasn't sure why just yet. Sophia was three degrees of separation from me and seeking her permission was a potential tedium of Chinese whispers.

I waited.

It was only days later when I awoke, soon finding myself with my ritual morning coffee, *and oddly*, opening my journal. The vortex pulled me in and I immediately began writing. Insight after insight, the pages filled with a story that wasn't mine. It expressed the pain of a life where joy and love had been lost to a patterned belief that love had to be earned, *and if it was earned*, it would be delivered empty through its measure. It was a tale of unworthiness, of being undeserving. Sadly, it was that familiar universal story of feeling unloved, told again and all too often.

With our souls connected, I gained perspective on Sophia's pain. I witnessed her hunger for love, her despondency, and I felt the lies and the heartbreak that had caused her to manifest this life-threatening problem. As I intuited all that was offered, I saw her, I heard her, and I sensed her. Scribing her messages, I filled with gratitude just to be able to sit at the edge of her mystery, aware that almost everything about her would remain completely unknown to me. There was an endless intrigue to her and it would continue to be guarded in the astonishing miracle of her Soul's uniqueness. If her truth could be known, it could only be captured in the essence of her telling.

"Divorce the story, marry the truth." – Anthony Robbins

Without a doubt, Sophia's story is important. Everybody's story is important. We give life meaning and we create meaning from life. Our stories reflect our ways of detailing and sharing our perceptions and perspectives about what we do, the encounters we have and our attitudes to life itself. We story through languaging – shading, shaping and colouring the depth and texture of our experiences... *and it all seems to matter.*

No offence, but in seeking to understand, be interested in only hearing your truth! A few embellishments won't hurt but as quickly as your story becomes an ocean of words, you are lost at sea and capsized all over again. If you want to save yourself, throw yourself the rope of truth that ties you to your life. In matters of life and death, I wonder what could be more important.

The key to the storytelling is to point to the truth. In the language and in the telling, we must reach in beyond our words – it's about the truth inside the story. What matters is that you really feel your experiences so your story telling becomes truth telling.

"We don't see things as they are, we see things as we are." – Anais Nin

Whatever story we share about our healing journey, scientists have drawn links between our emotions and our physical health. Perhaps what we might not be sure about is how we have each connected our dots.

Truth be told, no-one wants to believe they've created their own illness. It is useful to see that if we can create it, *we can un-create it*. The sad alternative is that if we choose to see disease *as something that happens to us*, we will not likely see ourselves as empowered beings that can undo the damage and return ourselves to homoeostasis.

If we accept that emotions, both positive and negative, impact on the state of our health, then disease and illness become our teachers, urging us to find ways to reconnect with ourselves at the core of who we are. This is an opportunity to understand the real cause of our disease, just as resistance serves only to prolong our suffering and move us further away from healing.

To restore our integrity, we must embrace all we have disowned about ourselves and accept the invitation to love those parts we cast out through judgment. In the reckoning, we must face our fears and find a new love and appreciation for all that we are, and see everything for what it is without condemnation for what it is not.

The way we think about things is important – thought is energy; our repeated thoughts give rise to our feelings and form our beliefs. Where our experiences leave our feelings unacknowledged, unexpressed or just plain unknown they stockpile into emotional patterns that get stored in the body, our subconscious mind, just waiting to be triggered. When we are set off, we often express our habitual thoughts and emotions without ever really knowing how we feel.

While we experience emotions physically, trapped negative emotions hold the potential to manifest as disease. Understanding our emotions means tapping into the body and journeying through our layers of experience, as if to map a new self-knowledge that recognises causation.

Awareness of what we are feeling is half the battle. From there, we can investigate the deeper meaning of how we have held our experiences. It is about identifying and understanding our repetitive thoughts, beliefs and emotions, to get to that place where we see what is unconsciously driving our dysfunction. By revealing false knowledge about who we think we are, we begin to release the internalised fears and self-judgment to find our way to a personal freedom that speaks to a truer version of who we are; self-acceptance and self-love are leverage for change.

"Out beyond ideas of wrongdoing and rightdoing there is a field. I'll meet you there." – Rumi

The truest nature of healing is mystical. If I can use any words, it is to say that healing happens in the space of possibilities, a space of pure awareness. I like to think of it as happening in the space that is *every-thing-ness* and *no-thing-ness* all at once. It is a space we rarely ever think of, or even notice, like when we are neither inhaling nor exhaling.

As a process, healing is a transformation that occurs instantaneously as if in a 'no time' space, held in the purest energy as if cupped by the hands of god not personified. The only thing I can liken it to is an epiphany – that moment of realisation inside another moment when we just get it.

The Operation

When I first learned of Sophia's tumour, I had been given its description: a small mass lodged between the two hemispheres of the brain, about eight centimetres long with some small tendrils; surgical intervention recommended. Weeks went by until I got a call to say her surgery had been suddenly moved up on the calendar; it was already underway. The growth had proliferated; it was alive. And it was killing her.

My morning dash was from the phone to a makeshift operating theatre in my lounge room! I scrubbed in as I faced east to do the usual invocation to all of my masters, guides and helpers – this time it was with a focused, almost willful intent and I called in extra help. After gaining Sophia's permission, I proceeded to cut her head open, the cut twice as long as I had known the growth to be. Oh! My mind tussled for a moment, thinking I had made my first surgical error. But I had to let that go. I had to focus on what I was seeing.

Surgery was demanding—precise, intense. Before long I was sweating. I worked with great care to remove the tumour. It was big, almost three times the size I'd been told. The mass had gained a firm hold on the corpus callosum between the left and right hemispheres and its tendrils had grown into every crevasse that barely offered an opening, trailing like roots of a tree.

As I etched out the growth with my blade, I intentionally though silently spoke to Sophia. I fed the journal entries back to her in affirmations and messages of healing; I now understood why telepathy was all that was needed. In other moments I chanted, as if singing to her.

When all was done, I thanked those who had entered to share my theatre and I acknowledged Sophia's courage as I smiled at her. I knew she was alive.

There is no right answer, no single prescription, as to how to heal. On a day to day level we make practical choices and take action. At a mystical level, we might hold to a power greater than ourselves and simply call it faith or hope.

Healing is not about fixing; it's not about something being wrong with us, or being broken. And it's not about stopping or masking symptoms, or removing bits that shouldn't be there. Quick fixes like medication address symptoms only to ignore the underlying signs of discontent. Medicine bypasses causation. But disease doesn't care what doctors think or what we choose to swallow – it shouts at us to pay attention. *Pay attention or you might pay with your life!*

And don't be fooled—during the process of healing, the very idea of taking time for ourselves is often lost in a slew of activities. Some choices like massage, meditation and yoga may offer definite therapeutic benefits, but others—like having a facial or getting our hair done – are little more than feel-good strategies that distract us from getting down and dirty with those mortal fears that threaten our very existence.

It is critical to listen to the body, to heed its warnings and to answer to its calling. But to answer fully and completely is a demanding inward journey. Truth telling is about getting inside the real pain, not the effects of the pain. The true energy of healing is about feeling your feelings, moving beyond the egoic story of lies that you have believed about yourself for too long, and getting to the truth that re-ignites and inspires life.

The energy of healing is ultimately a process of the individuated self finding its way back into the nurturing space of an unconditional love that offers an antidote for all we have experienced, real or imagined. It is our call to look beyond the symptoms and finally see what has caused us to feel the way we do and to undo the lies of those false and unloving programs that were installed at the time of our first emotional wounding. Healing is that time when we have to stand up and face our real fears, an invitation to know the self and to heal those wounds, emotion by emotion, layer by layer.

Just as an individual's unique expression of their biology, psychology, emotionality and spirituality contributes to creating disease or illness, the personal remedy that serves to holistically undo the damage and restore the individual to health might remain equally unknown.

"In every nation there are wounds to heal, in every community there is work to be done, in every heart there is the power to do it." – Marianne Williamson

The key to healing is awareness. The challenge is in making the unconscious conscious. And if the manifestation of disease, serious or otherwise, is a wake-up call, what are we waking up to? As complicated as we can possibly make our lives, simplicity remains the cornerstone. Healing requires one simple thing: love.

Healing is all about loving yourself. It is about the intention to heal, about giving yourself permission to be in the world and to live the life you were granted. The essence of allowing is lodged in the truth of your being, and all that is you and greater than you beckons you to surrender.

While there are those who seem to have some idea of how to love themselves, we are all still learning. Many of us were never shown, and most were certainly not encouraged. But we are now in a time that is calling upon us to operate from a whole-hearted consciousness. To honour ourselves we must be conscious of ourselves, of our experiences, and of our ways of being in the world. And in all ways, we must seek to do this through our heart and soul.

When we can bring our own story to its knees, we can move forward to consciously create more of the life we came to live. It is true of paradox that if we cannot know the darkness, we cannot see just how brightly we can shine; this is our wholeness.

As we choose to emerge from the darkness of our disowned humanity, in case you weren't really living before, illness invites you by asking, *"Do you really want to live now?"* At least it is honest with us.

If you accept the invitation, healing is only ever a decision away.

The Healing

A couple of days after the surgery, my one degree of separation called to share the surgeon's findings with me. Snap! It was a blueprint and I really had seen it. But something else got me. As it was recounted, Sophia was in recovery and the doctor asked her what day it was. He then asked her name and despite not knowing anyone by my name, she answered, *"Robyn"*. Something whipped through me as I put my hand over my mouth with a silent gasp of *oh my God!* My eyes welled—*we had been in communication* and although I thought I already knew that, this was my paradoxical moment of knowing that I knew nothing, and-but now knowing that the mystery that had brought us together was forever so real. There is no degree of separation in oneness. I was astounded.

That part of me that wondered for some time what was so important to Sophia that she had to go to so much trouble to look at it through a brain tumour, finally realised that the whole point was for me to reflect on why I had chosen my path and all of its manifestations as my healing journey.

Whatever her answer, it was for Sophia to know. I knew

that much. I was happy knowing that our soulful meeting had taken place in the mysterious intelligence of the universe. We had shared something and we would remain connected as we both moved on with our Soul's journeys.

"Who would you be without your story?" – Byron Katie

Sophia's story is a story about the intrinsic nature of the choices we make. If the paradox of life can offer us any insight that is served by the nature of wholeness that is paradox itself, then we can reveal the simplicity with which we are invited to life – to love, to be love, to live love.

There was really only one thing to be shared after all. It was a message for Sophia, as much as it is a message for me and for you. It is the simplest and most profound response to all of those universal stories of not feeling good enough, of feeling unlovable and in so many ways, of fearing life itself...

Love heals... And you are here to remember that you are love.

Inside the truth, the paradox of story and its ocean of pregnant words just disappear. Like I said, it's not about the story; it's about what's inside the story. And your life is about what's inside you.

"All matters are matters of the self." – Robyn James

I have learned that what we think matters and I have learned that how we feel matters. What matters most is finding our way to realising our own truth.

What's your inside story?

About the Author

ROBYN JAMES

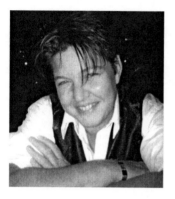

Robyn James is the founder of Inside Potential, an education-oriented holistic healing practice based in Brisbane, Australia. While she has one foot planted in the field of energy healing and the other firmly kicking about in personal growth and development, this empath describes her contribution and services as being at the crossroads where emotional healing meets personal empowerment.

As a passionate devotee of the self-healing road, Robyn has dedicated more than two decades to the field of metaphysical health and illness and she now shares her path to inspire others to see their own value and to feel empowered so they can realise their own potential. In clearing the path to living an extraordinary life, it has become far less about what's 'out there' and far more about what's on the inside... healing is simply about becoming more aligned with our authentic self and learning that the key is self-love.

Perhaps you will join Robyn on the ride to empower the healer within you. It can be quite a journey, so remember to share on the path... we are after all, just walking each other home.

Connect with Robyn via email to insidepotential@gmail.com and enjoy inspiring updates at Inside Potential on Facebook at https://www.facebook.com/insidepotential or connect and introduce yourself via LinkedIn – au.linkedin.com/in/robynjamesinsidepotential … and finally, visit the developing website at www.insidepotential. com.au.

Namaste!

Chapter 18

Vibrate Energy Healing into Your Life

By Laura Hackel

Things were about to change. 2002 was the year my understanding of the word "healing" was totally expanded. Up until then, I only considered the word appropriate to describe the literal healing of a physical body. Here's what happened.

At 37, I "had everything"; thriving traditional career, loving husband, three awesome kids, a house, a car and financial security. I specifically worked towards these things because I thought they would make me happy. What I found, however, was that after years of pouring myself into work and family, I was increasingly left with an empty feeling inside.

Don't get me wrong, I had moments of contentment, but they were fleeting and I found myself starting to develop a deep sense of hopelessness. I would ask myself, "Is this all there is to life?" I knew, somewhere deep inside that there was more to life and that's when a healing journey opened up for me.

What I now hold to be true is that healing is anything that shifts us into our own inner brilliance, the brilliance we are as we enter this world.

We are born into this world with strengths and gifts and as we go through life, we often make decisions – consciously or unconsciously – to ignore our gifts, downplay our strengths and even hide big pieces of ourselves. Often, we hide our gifts so effectively; we may never even know we have them. In essence, we are covering up our own inner brilliance.

My healing journey started the moment I decided there must be more to life and set about to find fulfillment. The first door that opened for me was Yoga. By practicing just twice a week I started breathing more and could literally feel space open up in my life. It helped me to realize that it was time to leave my corporate job of 17 years. Soon after, a close friend recommended a personal development program that gave me the tools to think about my life differently. From there, life opened up door after door for me including a strong calling to rediscover my repressed artistic side. I became a potter, started working with an energy healer, became a Shaman and eventually realized that my purpose here on this planet is to raise the vibration of individuals, groups, and the planet as a whole. These days, I wake up feeling grateful that I am living MY best life.

Let's talk a little more about vibration and its importance to healing. We know everything on the planet has a vibration, including each individual. As we go through life, there are some situations that expand our vibrations (feelings of self-love, confidence, trust in ourselves) and some experiences that lower vibration (feelings of shame, anger, sadness). It is not the feelings themselves that cause our vibration to drop, it is how we make ourselves wrong for our feelings that allow lower vibrations to work their way into our vibrational field and overstay their welcome.

Our vibration can stay lower for just a few hours, or it can get stuck in a lower level vibration for years. When our vibration is in a lower state we can not be our fully expressed, brilliant selves in the world.

Try a quick exercise with me:

Close your eyes *and recall a time this past week that you were frustrated, hurt, sad, angry or ashamed.*

Now think about how much time you spent in this place. How many people did you tell about your hurt, anger or frustration? How long did you spend in that feeling? *When you are done, imagine that there is an imaginary big hole in the earth on the right side of your body. Imagine letting the energy of those feelings drain into the hole.*

Now, **close your eyes** and think about something great that happened in the last week.

It might be as simple as a glimpse of the first flowers of

spring or the way the snow crystals formed on a tree branch, or as complex as a new baby or important life milestone.

Whatever it is, ask yourself how much time did you allow yourself to spend in this feeling? How many people did you tell about this feeling for a total of how much time? *When you are done, breathe that feeling into the area around your heart.*

Which feeling did you stay in longer? For most of us, it isn't even close, we spend more time in the lower vibrational energies like anger, sadness and fear. While the expanded energy of happiness comes in and goes easily, the lower energies can stay with us for a lifetime.

So, if healing is the journey of shifting into your own inner brilliance, the way to do that is to continually expand your vibration. Higher or expanded vibrations allow lower vibrational energies to be released from our energy fields and our physical bodies. As your vibrations rise, more possibilities open up for you as your inner brilliance shines out in the world and you feel a deep sense of connectedness and contentment.

Here are a few very easy ways to raise your vibration:

Movement: Stuck energy resembles a person who can't get off the couch. When you get up and move it around (dance like no one is watching, run in place, just move), the energy can literally shift with your movements.

Sound: If you are having a low energy moment, clap your

hands all around you several times and notice if you feel lighter. Or grab a rattle and some maracas and incorporate them into your dance to really shake up your energy. Try putting on music or singing your favorite song. The vibration in the music or song can clear stuck energy.

Thoughts: Surround yourself with thoughts that expand and serve you. When you are sending positive thoughts out to the universe, the universe responds by helping your thoughts become reality (the same happens with negative thoughts too, by the way).

While there are many ways to heal, one thing they all have in common is that the energy of healing is completely aligned with the energy of love. You see, the place where many of us go off track is that over time, we lose our ability to love ourselves. The more off track we get, the more healing we need to access our own brilliance.

Think about a two-year-old child. Their love of themselves is palpable. They don't naturally make judgments about whether they are good or bad and whether they deserve to be loved. They love themselves and everything around them unconditionally and they expect to be loved back.

As that same child grows up, they experience conditional love and judgment by others which has them start to judge themselves and step away from the self-love they were born with.

Our lack of self-love leads to pain in our bodies. What I have learned over the years is that the source of our physical pain shows up in our energy fields first. If we can clear the energy early enough, we can spare ourselves much physical discomfort.

Let's do another exercise.

Close your eyes and breathe. As you are breathing, check in with your body to see if it is experiencing any tightness or pain. If you are, note where.

Every time we swallow our uncomfortable, negative feelings or emotionally disconnect from others because it is too painful, we are storing low vibration energy in our energy fields. This low energy can get "stuck" both in our energy field and our physical bodies and lowers our vibration. When something is wrong in your physical body, you take action to correct it. Whether it's changing your eating habits, getting a massage, or visiting a doctor, you know that you don't want to live with pain in your body.

For example, whenever I have a sharp pain in my left knee, I know that what is coming up for me is something to do with expressing my needs with my family of origin. Let me explain:

I grew up with three brothers and each of us are less than two years apart. As a child, I often did not have a choice about what we were going to do. We all took swimming lessons or we all played tennis because it was the only way to mange it logistically. I made an unconscious decision not to rock the boat to keep peace in the family. In doing so, I disconnected from the part of me that could identify and express my needs. Although this made the family waters smoother as a child, when I fast forward 20 years to being married with three children and an inability to identify or express my needs I realize the impact of that unconscious decision.

What I have since learned is that each time I repressed my needs, I was unconsciously creating low vibrational blocks in my left knee and my knee would literally hurt. After 30 plus years of stuffing the energetic hurt of not having my needs met, I found a book that was key to my understanding of what was happening. "The surprising purpose of anger: Beyond Anger Management: Finding the Gift", describes how all forms of anger (from annoyance to rage and everything in between) are really a sign that you have a need that is not being met.

Close your eyes and recall the last time you were angry or frustrated, or annoyed. What was happening around you? What need did you have that was not being met in the moment?

Here's where it can get kind of tricky. Most of the time you don't look at yourself and say "Why didn't I meet that need that I wasn't even aware that I had?"

Instead, most often we say, "He made me angry" or "She isn't supporting me" or "He doesn't appreciate me".

In reality, what you are REALLY angry about is that you are not supporting or appreciating yourself. But, you can't see it that way so you blame others for your upset. Not pretty is it? The great news is, that you can do something about it. You can't change what the other person is doing, but you can change how you think about what the other person is doing and take responsibility for getting your own needs met.

Let's take an example here. One year, I was frustrated (a form of anger) at my husband because my birthday party was not what I wanted it to be. I was hurt that the party didn't reflect what I wanted. After I got over myself, I started to wonder how he got the ideas for the party. I realized that he had asked me several times what I wanted *and I didn't know what I wanted so I never answered the question clearly.*

This was the catalyst for my breakthrough around seeing that I didn't have the skill to identify and express what I wanted (yet!). I had to think of a girlfriend of mine who was much more aware and communicative of her needs, and ask myself "What would Di want?" From there I would get five or six ideas and then I could figure out which one (s) appealed to me.

It was a tedious process for sure, but it actually built a bridge so that I can now connect directly to my wants and needs. While it seemed to take years, I had to remember that I spent 35 years ignoring my needs so getting back in touch with them over two years was actually an amazing achievement.

The next time you experience physical pain, consider thanking the pain for giving you a clue that you might be suppressing a need or an emotion that wants to be heard. It's also a signal that it's time to raise your vibration.

Step one of healing is to decide that you are ready to embark on a journey to fully express your gifts and greatness in the world. Don't forget to breathe here and remember, you don't have to do it all at once, it will evolve over time and the universe will support you on this journey. There are many ways to release lower vibrational energy that you don't want to carry around anymore.

Energy Healing Tips:

1) Protect yourself energetically every day. Whether you use my favorite protection "I am the light, the light is within me, the light moves through out me, the light surrounds me, the light protects me, I AM the light." Or imagine yourself inside of bubble filled with white light that allows in loving energy and stops any energy that doesn't serve you from entering your energy field.

2) Keep Your Environment Clear. The energy from your own thoughts and the thoughts of everyone who enters your space get stored in your space and will stay there until it is cleared. You can easily clear out space using smudge sticks or clearing spray for a fresh start. Simply hold the intention for any energy that is not there to serve your or your family to be released as you smudge or spray the room in a clockwise direction. You can buy smudge spray (Murray and Lannon Florida Water) on Amazon and place it in an atomizer for easy use.

3) Become a Detective. Start looking for the connection between your thoughts and feelings and the events that happened. Dive into what makes you angry and see what your unmet needs are. Commit to meeting those needs.

4) Develop as strong practice of self-love. Identify what you need every day and make sure you allow time to receive it. It could be a workout, a walk in nature, a quiet few minutes for yourself or time to read a book or take a bath, If you are a beginner at this, just pick one thing that's important to you and schedule and make the time to do it each day for a week. If someone else asks for that time, politely decline. For me it's a workout, time spent outside (could even be with my laptop), quiet time for meditation and reflection, and time to work on creative projects.

5) Develop a practice that supports raising your vibration. Try:

a. Dancing, swimming, bicycling

b. Yoga, at least three different types to see which ones work for you

c. Acupuncture

d. Making an appointment with an energy healer

e. Listening to healing music

f. A Crystal Bowl Healing

When you heal yourself, you also heal those around you.

Your energy of living in your inner brilliance opens the doors for others to live in theirs.

I have learned there are many ways to release lower vibrational energy that is not serving you anymore. One of my favorite ways is with the Crystal Bowls.

Each bowl is made of quartz crystal and you lay down and relax while I play them to vibrate at a frequency so high that stuck energy is released from your field.

By declaring up front what you are ready to release (old stuck energy) and what you want to invite in (new, expansive energy), you will be raising or expanding you vibration to reveal more of your fully expressed, brilliant self.

After a crystal bowl session, people tell me that they have:

- Started to see a stressful situation in a whole new light that allowed them to step in and take action

- Felt heavy, stuck energy being yanked away from their hearts

- Accessed a deep space of connection and self –love

To hear the crystal bowls in action, visit her website and artfulhealings.com

Whatever method works for you, know that the path will open up for you as you go along.

Now open your eyes and experience the life that is waiting for you to claim it!

About the Author

LAURA HACKEL

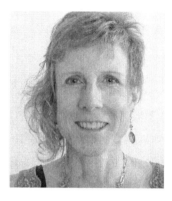

Laura is a vibrational energy healer and artist, wife, mother of three, writer, and bringer of light to this planet.

She can be found spending her days between her ceramics studio and her healing studio where she delights in helping people make a deeper connection to their soul and the wisdom of their souls and to experience the deep inner wisdom and beauty that exists in the layers, textures and patterns within.

Laura works her magic to help you raise your vibration and live the life you want by using her background as a corporate executive, her Shaman and energy healing training, her intuition and zest for life in general.

One of her favorite ways to clear out stuck energy and bring in high vibrational energy is by playing the crystal bowls for groups and events. Each Bowl is made of quartz crystal and you have lay down and relax as she coaxes beautiful sounds from them that vibrate at the exact frequency you need to first release what it blocking you and then bring in the energy of what you desire.

To hear the crystal bowls in action, visit her website at artfulhealings.com

Laura also makes amazing vibrational Healing Vessels. Each Healing Vessel is formed with her own hands, to facilitate vibrational shifting in both your home and life. There are many shapes and sizes to choose from; each is one of a kind, lovingly handcrafted and sure to shift the energy of any space. Each Healing Vessel is infused with Healing Energy.

To select the perfect healing vessel for you, visit artfulhealings.com. You can access her blog and event schedule at artfulhealings.com. Or you can connect on facebook at facebook/artful.healings.

Chapter 19

Healing the Veil So Love Can Emerge

By Connie Viveros

How would it feel to discover you've been living behind a veil? An invisible screen preventing you from realizing a pure love that could heal you whenever and wherever you needed it? A barrier to reaching your fullest potential and in fact what is standing directly between you and your most magnificent self? What if it were possible to heal or even remove this veil so that your own magnificent expression of this pure love became a living reality rather than an impossible dream?

My own decades-long journey of self discovery has led me to come face-to-face with this veil and devote myself to healing it in order to realize that pure love in a deeper, more profound way, every day. What is this invisible veil, anyway?

Why is it there, hiding this healing love that we all long for? It can take many forms, but primarily it's made up of our limiting beliefs. Rooted in our shadow and kept intact by self-loathing, it's woven through with our own particular set of limiting beliefs, which could sound like this – love is not possible, I don't deserve happiness, I'm not good enough, I'll never have everything I dream of. Sound familiar? Your veil may have a different pattern to it, but whatever it looks like, it's convincing, powerful, and probably unconscious. Its job is to block us from our light, our truth, our Love, and it's very good at it. But it's not indestructible. I've come to understand that we can heal this veil and step into the light by accepting and loving the dark. It might seem counterintuitive, but accepting and loving all of ourselves, our darkness as well as our light, opens the veil to what's behind it.

And love is what's behind the veil. Not the kind of love that is romantic or sexual, or even the type of love that is felt between family and friends. The love to which I am referring, the love on the other side of the veil is agape love–pure, unconditional, Divine Love. This love that lives behind the veil, underneath the buried treasure of your shadows, is God's perfect love.

Many of us don't even recognize that our ultimate purpose on this planet is to be an expression of agape or Divine Love, and to endow everything we do with this pure form of God's Spirit. Endowing everything with this Love actualizes Divine Spirit in you. Imagine love manifesting fully inside of you–what would or could you become?

To understand the spiritual path, it's important to begin at the beginning—to realize that we were all originally light and that we dwelled in the cosmos of Spirit/God/agape love.

We voluntarily asked to be here, to incarnate at this time, this place, and God granted our request and we came into the material universe. We gradually became enmeshed in denser and denser dimensions, with the veil growing thicker and thicker through our ego's experiences, until we found ourselves embodied on this small planet, far away from our spiritual home. All the while, we've had a deep (though sometimes unconscious) desire to pierce the veil, and get back to the business of our soul's journey of permanently uniting with our Higher Self. This integration, the removal of the veil, is both the journey and the healing that needs to occur as we become love, the I AM presence—so that we can heal and return to our eternal nature!

So how do we go about doing this? How do we pierce or dissolve the veil so we can return to this ever-present, continually vibrating existence of love? To begin, we must first understand our unique mission, our divine purpose here at this time. One clue is that your mission is often tied to your passion. So first you must ask yourself, What am I passionate about? As we honor our passions, we can also get clues to our mission by developing our God-given talents. We embark on a journey of uncovering our divine purpose by noticing and honoring who we already are.

Let me share a little bit about my process of uncovering my own mission as a spiritual healer. For some years now I've coached people in the area of healing emotional wounds and traumas, helping them overcome limiting beliefs in areas of their life where they feel stuck and unable to move forward. Over the past few years, my coaching sessions have been increasingly filled with an energy of healing light and warmth. I've felt profoundly moved by the presence of this unconditional love or energy in these sessions, felt even while conducting appointments over the phone. I've been blessed to be a part of many powerful transformations in people's lives, and this has been deeply gratifying and meaningful to me.

A little over three years ago, I experienced a technique of spiritual healing called 'channeling.' It was profound for me, and I have been studying and practicing it ever since, devoting hundreds of hours to my own personal learning and practice. I've also slowly integrated channeling into my coaching practice. The integration has been spontaneous and organic, rather than as a result of a specific intent to incorporate the technique into my sessions.

During these sessions, I and my clients have been deeply affected by this powerful spiritual healing. Through devoted study and practice I've now become a 'Master Channel.' Thanks to this newfound practice, my own passion, or life's true purpose and mission, has been revealed to me, in great detail, and I have discovered in me a whole new Divine path, a way for me to uniquely express God's love in this lifetime. And guess what? To my utter amazement, as I continue to pierce my own veil of limitation, and support others in doing that for themselves, our souls reveal that we're all much bigger (and better!) than we ever dreamed or imagined!

But prior to becoming a Master Channel, I didn't know what my purpose was. I just knew that I needed to find it. That became my mission. All I knew about it was that it had something to do with a 'mission for God', and all I needed was find out how to be a unique expression of Divine Love in this world. Above all else I craved knowing my life, the answer to "why am I here?" – in finding myself, my talents, my calling and my service to life.

Each day during my young adulthood I would meditate and study those things, teachings, courses that would lead me closer to the understanding of my life's mission. My desire to love my life and who I was supposed to become led me, even compelled me, on a deep journey of self discovery that continues to this day!

My dedication paid off. When I first witnessed the person I am destined to become, I had the realization that this person already existed inside of me. I was fascinated to find that the beautiful person I so longed to be was actually living within me. I also discovered that this truly beautiful person was buried deep beneath my conscious awareness – behind a veil!

For years I had wanted to be a good person, to walk the spiritual talk, to believe in myself, and live a life that mattered. I admired and looked up to anyone who was living a life enmeshed in their passion. I wanted to wake up every morning knowing that I was living my life to its fullest. The day I came face to face with my authentic self I was shocked. I was shocked because at the time I believed that the self I thought I was supposed to be would come via some Divine intervention, some message from an archangel bearing special gifts for me from beyond – much like the biblical stories of Mother Mary or even Moses! To my amazement, however, she did not come from outside of me, nor did she make herself known through discarding certain aspects of myself which I found unnecessary. She came from accepting myself exactly as I was in that moment...flawed and fabulous, temperamental and easy going, lovable and unlovable!

What I understood that it was not my purpose to get rid of everything I felt was wrong or bad about myself, but in fact just the opposite. It was my job to take my most human self and transform her into my most extraordinary self through becoming whole. The veil was pulled back to reveal to me that my most Divine self lay hidden in my most human self, and from this place of integrating the two, I could enliven a life of my dreams.

It was in this moment that I discovered the Self I was longing for was hiding behind the veil, buried deep within my humanity. I finally knew what true love really felt like. For the first time ever, I loved my WHOLE ENTIRE SELF! This feeling of complete love came without conditions. A love without restriction, a love that holds the most compassionate and loving thoughts rather than critical, self-berating thoughts. A love that is filled with caring for oneself rather than self loathing. To see this "spiritual blueprint" of my life was an extraordinary and reassuring experience. With the veil pulled back I was completely exposed, and completely in love! The love I discovered brought me to experience a new reality. I found the courage to reclaim my most authentic self, understood with ease what my purpose and my passion were, and connected to my deep desire to help heal humankind.

Our culture is driven by our ego's needs. This drives us to want to be important, to be recognized as wonderful, great, or admirable. Yet this is driven by our shadow, hiding from us life's true meaning, which is love. Love is what we live for, what we long for, what we want to give and to receive, no matter who we are. In our culture, we tend to think of love as something separate from us, as though it isn't something we have. Yet love is our true nature. Love is mighty and powerful enough to awaken us, transform us, and even bring healing. Through love we receive understanding, mercy, joy, and forgiveness. Through love we have what it takes to truly meet our needs, and give to others. Through love we feel worthy and valid. Through love we serve a higher purpose and unite in a higher calling.

You deserve to live a life of love and to experience the healing quality of the most beautiful love you've ever imagined. You are the Light, and as such you are pure, divine, purposeful and deserving. By bringing your darkness to the light, and claiming your light, you will begin to dissolve the veil, growing and strengthening your own spiritual healing power.

The Light will move upon the darkness. It's not the other way around, though often when we're caught in a dark place, it feels like the light is far away from us and we feel powerless. Yet, it is the Light which actually carries supreme power. Light has the power to trump all darkness. Light is greater than darkness. It's the remover of darkness. This is the process of healing. And it works. But in order for this to work we must expose our darkness to the Light, pierce the veil, pull back the curtain and allow what's behind to emerge – absolute love, the kind of love you will never forget.

The experience of Love in this form will grow as you take time to heal pain in your life. As you release the negative false beliefs that tell you that you are somehow wrong for being who you are, you begin to poke holes in this veil, exposing rays of Divine love that will keep you returning again and again until one day, it is dissolved for good. As you open up to more compassion, forgiveness, acceptance and love, your life becomes filled with true abundance – an overwhelming feeling that who and what you are is enough, that you are deeply deserving and dearly loved. Only from this place of a fully tended consciousness can your true purpose flourish, as the road rises up to meet you and deliver the life of your dreams.

Commit to loving yourself in every way. It's time you received unlimited love from yourself, all the time. Why not? Start with forgiving yourself for everything you've ever done that you regret. Then move on toward acting with kindness toward yourself and cherishing yourself as the precious piece of gold that you are. Lift the veil. You'll be glad you did.

Here are a few suggestions and practices you can begin that will help you begin lifting the veil, and opening up to the healing power of Divine, unconditional love.

Stop comparing yourself to others. You are not supposed to be like anyone else. You are the only one who can be you. Your perspectives, gifts and value are exclusively yours. You are a unique expression of the Divine.

Allow yourself to be where you are. Allow yourself to freely feel whatever you are feeling, without judging it or judging yourself for feeling it. Let go of the story you have created around it and just be with each feeling. All of emotions and feelings are of value, and want to be felt fully. This can only be done when you let go of your resistance to feeling it, which is kept in place by the story and the judgment you have around it.

Step outside the paradigm of limited love and imagine yourself within a realm of nothing but love. Begin to imagine a place where Love is everywhere! And you're in the middle of it.

Decide once and for all that **you are completely deserving of this love**. Let it fill you up, beginning with your heart, and expanding into all parts of your body.

Be true to yourself. Live your life doing what feels right to you, not what someone else thinks you should do. It's ok to listen to advice, but in the end, make the decision that feels best for you. Get in the habit of pleasing yourself, and engage in activities that bring you joy.

About the Author

CONNIE VIVEROS

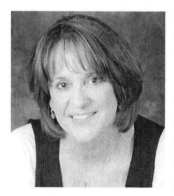

Connie Viveros is a Master Integrative Life Coach who helps people find more meaning in their lives and overcome the often unexplained emotional pain that keeps them from experiencing life's true joy. Connie is professionally trained as a Master Integrative Coach through the Ford Institute for Transformational Training, and is certified in multiple Integrative Coaching programs. She is also a Certified Passion Test Facilitator and a Master Spiritual Channel and Intuitive.

Prior to coaching, Connie spent many successful years as a corporate professional while devoting decades to her own spiritual growth and personal exploration. She started her coaching business in 2008 to help others deal with the sometimes overwhelming prospect of authentically changing their lives. If you have a desire to create lasting change in some area of your life–relationships, body image, work or career– Connie can help you unlock what has been holding you back, and transform pain into possibility to achieve just about anything you desire. If you are willing to create your greatest life, experience profound relationships, and follow your dreams then she would love to coach you to success.

Connie offers a wide range of programs and services, from individual coaching to seminars and workshops, as well as keynote speeches. To contact her, please visit her website www.ConnieViveros.com.

Chapter 20

Trust Energy to Heal Ancient Pain

BY ERICA GLESSING

Healing for me shows up when the trust in the light out-weighs and overcomes the darkness. The darkness is insidious and creeps back into my life, in the form of those who deliver judgment, unkindness, and destruction. And yet, the darkness cannot exist in the light.

The beauty happens for me when I choose healing as the path I stand in, and the path I share with others so that they may also heal and tune into the being of light that I believe each person is, underneath and behind everything else that we are.

Healing may require an intense discipline of me, so that I can allow the light and follow the truth and the energy of myself.

The truth is healing.

The truth is wellness.

The truth is abundance.

The truth is love.

Everything else is a lie. When I surround myself with the light, I am so blessed to be surrounded by smiling, warm, loving people in my life.

And I'm learning to reach into the places where I've let myself be the darkness, and invite the light to heal and resolve wounds that I carried into this world in my very cellular memory from other lifetimes and other worlds. Within my cells, the very universe lies.

When I don't know how to clear out the unhappiness, I'm shifting out of healing and into places that are calling for healing in my life. I can call upon my body to give me answers, and I can call upon source energy to bring wisdom forth. In the listening to the quiet voice within my soul, the doorway to healing opens and my mind and body feel free again.

I keep wondering if at some point I will feel healed, from all of the wounds I've suffered in my life. I keep wondering if there is this place of nirvana that I might suddenly one day reach where my heart and mind and body are whole again.

Bits of broken pieces of me lay scattered along my lifeline. I chose a difficult road this lifetime. I chose a family that judged my body so viciously for so many years, that family events were a trauma to be survived. Each year at Easter and Christmas I would go see family, waiting for them to comment on my weight or my body, or how awful I looked to them.

Now most of that family has died, and I'm healthy, so it is time to let go of all of that. Being of a body that is Italian and curvy, I basically was wrong in my slender family, and whatever I created, wrote, generated, or became was most certainly not ever going to please the people in my life. They were ashamed of me and often I would not get invited to events because of the embarrassment they felt looking at me. I remember going to my brother's wedding and hearing "He has a sister?" by friends whom had never seen or heard of me.

I recognize that we choose our parents, and I did choose some fantastic writers as parents. My skills are third generation and I'm blessed with not only writing skills, but television production skills, radio production skills, and book publishing skills. My son is so cute when he says "Mom, you have mad skills. You can do anything." That family gave me a lot of my gifts by way of genetics and lineage.

Healing for me came in the allowance of myself and the recognition of that which gives me joy. Healing comes each day when I let it in.

As I write, I wonder, what have I healed from in my life that could give courage to another? And I wonder, what healing energy can I give to others by my very being?

A Darker, Younger Choice

I'm pretty sure I won't understand why I chose to marry someone with whom I was so poorly matched, even in years, when I'm standing on the gates between this life and the next. I could guess my 30-year-old self chose him because he was a match on some levels, but truly as I survive the divorce I am not clear why he ended up in my life. So being married to him carries with it no happy memories. I look back at that time in my life, and there are no highlight reels. I survived.

He drank and I woke up drenched in his incontinence for most of the time we were together. He smoked and I can still smell the putrid tobacco smell that surrounded him. He would lose body control and so everything around him smelled like his urine, including the mattress and the couches that I replaced a few times each year. I replaced the carpet and the couches in the family room but the smell would permeate.

I laugh when people say "remember the good times" and with the exception of the children, there weren't any. So, I just lived asleep in my emotions for 17 years until one morning I woke up. It was July 7, 2011. I woke with the awareness of being done. He had "leaked" all over me, and the bedding. At the hotel where we were staying, it was quite booked, and there were no more blankets, I had no blankets. So I was freezing, and I said, I don't have to be married to him anymore. And that was it. This huge joy overcame my entire being.

Oh, that was a beautiful day. That was the beginning of the

greatest healing and the welcoming of myself back into my body. My spirit was overjoyed to the point where I would just laugh and smile and sing and dance to myself.

I am so joyful to be myself again. I re-discovered joy at age 50. I became reborn and experienced healing regardless of the past, and regardless of the pain and misery that at some level I chose to endure.

This healing of my spirit is most certainly not complete. I wake up days when I forget my beauty, yet again. I forget that my spirit is more than my physical anyhow, and I forget that part of me that which is infinite.

And then again, I wake up fresh and wondering what life will bring me today. Ideas and projects and books are always being born within my heart, and I yearn to keep birthing beautiful books and to keep appreciating all of the beautiful people who have made themselves present in my life.

I am so blessed to have creation move within me each day—that place where life begets more life, and joy begets more joy. I wake up each day with eyes wide open, wondering how miracles of creation will be born inside of me and how I can encourage miracles to be created with everyone I meet.

This new fresh love and new fresh eyes on the world are the true miracle of healing for me. As love courses through me and love opens me up to more vulnerability, I am letting the healing take place.

I am so joyful I did not wait longer to leave the brutality of what being married was for me.

Many of the authors in this book have taught me about healing. Donna LaBar is one of the authors who shares "if you scratch your arm, will it heal?" and you say "yes," it will. By simply allowing healing, healing will happen.

So as I move my pain and my memories out of the way, I let in the light. I let in the love. I let in the places where the sunshine can warm me, and the ocean can roar near me. This love of life and love of each and every waking moment is the birthright I am now allowing in.

The Truth is Healing

As I stand in the truth, the love, the light and the true being of me, I am present to all of the lies that I bought over time. The lies erode confidence, where truth gives strength and brings joy into my waking moments.

My gratitude for each and every author in this book is supreme. The healing you all bring will give wings to love, joy and light to soar.

My own journey is far from complete! I stand here in the light of my very being allowing myself to be a healing source for others. I am still learning my healer self, and I believe the awakening of this healing capacity that I have will guide me in the years to come.

I ask a lot of questions every morning.

What can life bring me today? What is possible today that I have never yet considered? What amazing miracle might show up today? What would my body like to experience today? Who should I connect with today? I just ask, and let the answers begin to form themselves in my life. I love when I ask for more than I have ever allowed to show up.

Will you allow healing to show up in your life? Invite this!

About the Author
ERICA GLESSING

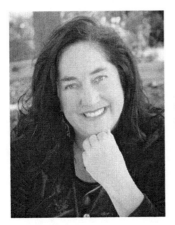

Erica Glessing is a dreamer, a bright writer, an editor, a publisher, a medium, an animal communicator, a mom, a happiness coach, and a loving spirit. You can find out more about Erica at www.EricaGlessing.com, www.Facebook.com/happinessquotations and feel free to friend her on Facebook or follow her on Twitter.

Her company, Happy Publishing, is dedicated to publishing the works of light bringers on the planet. The bestselling books Happy Publishing has released in 2015 so far include "The Energy of Happiness"; "The Energy of Receiving"; "The Energy of Expansion"; and "The Energy of Healing."

The End

About Happy Publishing

Happy Publishing is dedicated to supporting authors who wish to change the world. Happy Publishing has published more than 125 authors since its inception. Books released so far include:

The Energy of Healing (May, 2015)

The Energy of Happiness (2015)

The Energy of Receiving (2015)

Manifest Change (2014)

The Dreams of Mattie Fitch (2014)

Something About Sophia (2013)

Luxury Home Selling Mastery (2014)

Home Buying Mastery (2013)

Coming up in 2015:

The Energy of Creativity

I'm Having It

The Energy of Play

And what else is possible?

Erica Glessing is the CEO of Happy Publishing. Happy Publishing is under Ingram, the finest book distribution company on the planet today.

Erica is a third generation publisher, and second generation published author. She began writing professionally in 1984 as a news reporter. She has written *Prospect When You Are Happy* in 2007 and *Happiness Quotations: Gentle Reminders of Your Preciousness,* in 2011.

She works with writers to bring out the best in them. Happy Publishing was formed with the writer in mind. Email: HappyPublishing@gmail.com.

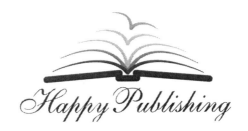

Happy Publishing

CPSIA information can be obtained
at www.ICGtesting.com
Printed in the USA
FFOW03n0159030216
20962FF